Neonatal and Early Onset Diabetes Mellitus

Ivana Rabbone • Dario Iafusco
Editors

Neonatal and Early Onset Diabetes Mellitus

From Pathogenesis to Novelty in Treatment

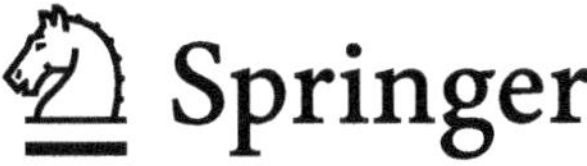

Editors
Ivana Rabbone
Division of Pediatrics
Department of Health Sciences
University of Piemonte Orientale
Novara, Italy

Dario Iafusco
Department of Woman, Child, and General and Specialistic Surgery
University of Campania Luigi Vanvitelli
NAPOLI, Napoli, Italy

ISBN 978-3-031-07010-5 ISBN 978-3-031-07008-2 (eBook)
https://doi.org/10.1007/978-3-031-07008-2

This Springer imprint is published by the registered company Springer Nature Switzerland AG
The registered company address is: Gewerbestrasse 11, 6330 Cham, Switzerland

Contents

Chapter 1
History of Neonatal Diabetes

Carla Bizzarri, Riccardo Schiaffini, and Ippolita Patrizia Patera

> *All cases that have come to my attention of youthful patients with diabetes living for many long periods of time have been hereditary.*
>
> *Elliott Proctor Joslin, 1934*

Neonatal diabetes mellitus (DM) has been usually defined as the onset of persistent hyperglycemia within the first 6 months of life [1]. Hyperglycemia in a neonate is not an uncommon occurrence, therefore, making the diagnosis of neonatal DM can be difficult [1–3]. Transient neonatal hyperglycemia is more common during the first 3–5 days of life and resolves within 2–3 days, but can persist up to 10 days. In preterm or small for gestational age babies, the prevalence of hyperglycemia can range from 25% to 75% [1]. For this reason, the terminology describing DM in the first year of life has been sometimes confusing, especially in early studies [3]. Although some patients present within the first 30 days of life (i.e., strictly defined neonatal period), infants most often show the onset of the disease within the first 6 months of life, and occasionally up to 12 months of age [2]. Therefore, the term neonatal DM, as it is now commonly used both in the literature and clinical settings, refers to patients up to 1 year of life who present with monogenic DM.

Supplementary Information The online version contains supplementary material available at https://doi.org/10.1007/978-3-031-07008-2_1.

C. Bizzarri (✉) · R. Schiaffini · I. P. Patera
Unit of Endocrinology and Diabetes, Bambino Gesù Children's Hospital, Rome, Italy
e-mail: carla.bizzarri@opbg.net; riccardo.schiaffini@opbg.net; ipatrizia.patera@opbg.net

I. Rabbone, D. Iafusco (eds.), *Neonatal and Early Onset Diabetes Mellitus*, https://doi.org/10.1007/978-3-031-07008-2_1

Most cases of neonatal DM present with intrauterine growth retardation (IUGR), failure to thrive, decreased subcutaneous fat, and low or undetectable C-peptide levels [1, 2]. This form of hyperglycemia has been also termed as "congenital" DM, in contrast with the rare forms of "acquired" autoimmune type 1 DM presenting within the first 6 months of life.

The earliest report on DM presenting in an infant was published in *1789* by Rollo [4].

Kitselle in *1852* [5] described his son who shortly after birth showed polydipsia, polyuria, failure to thrive, and glycosuria. This child died after a few months.

The second case, described in *1910* by Cuno [6], was a 15-day-old baby with glycosuria and hyperglycemia who died shortly after diagnosis. Atrophy of the pancreas was found at postmortem examination.

In *1926*, Ramsey [7] reported the case of a 4-week-old premature baby presenting with excessive appetite and thirst, glycosuria, and hyperglycemia. This baby appeared to recover completely in 6 weeks and showed a normal glucose tolerance 4 years later.

In *1931*, Lawrence and McCance [8] reported the case of an 18-day-old baby with gangrene of the leg who had glycosuria and a blood glucose level of 600 mg/dl. At 6 weeks of age, this child recovered spontaneously. These authors reviewed the existing literature and defined the diagnostic criteria of neonatal DM as cases with a suggestive clinical picture (polyuria, polyuria, wasting) with heavy glycosuria, even if hyperglycemia was not established, or (b) cases showing recurrent hyperglycemia (>200 mg/dl), even in the absence of specific symptoms. They pointed out that some of the previously published cases showed a rapid and complete DM remission, after a few weeks or months from the onset of the disease. They considered these cases to be unjustified and supposed that their hyperglycemia was related to the concomitant severe condition (mostly systemic infections and disorders of the central nervous system). We now know that sepsis, increased counter-regulatory hormones due to stress, parenteral glucose administration, and medications such as steroids and beta-adrenergic drugs represent common causes of hyperglycemia in preterm neonates (particularly infants with gestational age < 32 complete weeks). In critically ill preterm neonates, there is also evidence of reduced insulin secretion and relative insulin resistance. On the other hand, we currently know that some children with genetically confirmed forms of neonatal DM show a mild and transient course of the disease and need insulin therapy just for a few days. In a case series of 750 patients with DM diagnosed before 6 months of age, preterm children with and without a confirmed DM-causing mutation showed similar clinical characteristics, age of presentation, birth weight, and time to referral [1].

In *1932*, White [9] had already studied a large population of 750 patients with DM onset during childhood and reported that 16% of them were younger than 4 years at DM presentation, whereas the disease occurred before the age of 1 year in only 0.5%. Later studies confirmed a proportion of 7 infants out of 1430 children at DM diagnosis [4].

In *1935*, Lewis and Eisenberg [10] reported the case of a female baby who had otitis media and bullous impetigo and was found to have glycosuria and blood glucose levels between 280 and 520 mg/dl. In the same year, Limper and Miller [11] reviewed the case of a child with gangrene of the leg, glycosuria, and a blood glucose level of 952 mg/dl. Neither of these infants survived long, in spite of insulin therapy. At postmortem examination, congenital deficiency of the islet tissue was found in the first case; while acute degeneration of the islets was in the latter one. We can speculate that the first case [10] was affected by neonatal DM associated with pancreatic hypoplasia, while the second one [11] could represent the first report of insulitis in the context of a monogenic autoimmune neonatal diabetes.

In *1947*, Schwartzmann, Crusius, and Beirne [12] reviewed 57 cases with the onset of DM symptoms in the first year of life. They concluded that positive family history, infections, and disorders of the central nervous system, such as hydrocephalus or other brain malformations, were the main etiologic factors. Early symptoms were weight loss, dehydration, irritability, and/or "crystalline deposits on the diapers." Skin conditions, gangrene, cataract, infections of the respiratory tract, metabolic acidosis, and coma were common complications early after DM diagnosis. The most common findings at autopsy were atrophy of the pancreas, with a decrease in size and number of the islets of Langerhans, and fatty degeneration of the liver. Treatment was based on a diet approaching the normal one, supplemented with insulin and vitamins, as needed.

In *1962*, Hutchinson, Keay and Kerr [13] reviewed 11 cases of what they called "congenital temporary diabetes mellitus" and highlighted the peculiar clinical picture of severe dehydration and wasting at presentation. They stated: *"The literature of diabetes mellitus in infancy reveals a certain amount of confusion, largely attributable to the fact that the aetiology of diabetes remains unknown. It is well recognized that in adults the term diabetes mellitus includes more than one disease. It is perhaps insufficiently appreciated that the same is true of the infant. Two types can now be separated. In older infants insulin-sensitive diabetes mellitus with ketosis and acidosis necessitates the lifelong use of insulin, and it is not distinguishable from the common type of diabetes of later childhood and early adult life. There is, however, another type, with onset at or shortly after birth, which is also insulin-sensitive but is not accompanied by ketosis, and which appears to be capable of spontaneous recovery."* The authors noted that DM severity and duration of insulin dependency varied widely, but all patients responded to insulin, even if a wide variability of blood glucose levels was evident, with alternating hypo- and hyperglycemia. Differently from patients with type 1 DM, ketosis and metabolic acidosis were usually mild or absent. At that time, half-cream dried cow milk enriched with sucrose was usually used to feed and avoid hypoglycemia [13]. After the start of insulin therapy, most children grew rapidly and developed obesity and "moon face" appearance mimicking hypercortisolism. Steroid hormone levels were found normal or slightly increased. Psychomotor assessment showed global developmental delay, spastic paresis, and epilepsy in a significant proportion of cases. It is now well known that some forms of neonatal DM are primarily associated with brain malformations, psychomotor delay, and/or epilepsy. On the other hand, the high doses of insulin that were used at that time (more than 1 U/kg/dose of soluble human insulin every 3–6 h) had a rapid and remarkable anabolic effect, but probably the consequent alternation of severe hypoglycemia and hyperglycemia contributed not only to the development of obesity but also to the brain damage of these patients.

In *1995* [14], paternal uniparental isodisomy (UPD) of an imprinted region in the long arm of chromosome 6 was first described in children with transient neonatal DM, who usually showed remission of hyperglycemia in infancy (by 13–18 weeks of age), followed by DM recurrence in adolescence or adulthood in 50% of cases.

In *2002*, a crucial study by Iafusco et al. [15] highlighted that most DM cases with onset within 6 months from birth do not have an autoimmune pathogenesis. The clinical and genetic characteristics of 111 patients who received insulin within 12 months of life were studied. The epidemic curve of age at DM onset revealed two subsets of patients at a cutoff of 180 days. In the group with DM onset before 180 days ("early onset" permanent diabetes) the analysis of HLA heterodimers showed that 76% had a "protective" HLA genotype for type 1 DM, as compared to 11.9% of the "later onset" group. The distribution of HLA markers of susceptibility to type 1 diabetes in the "early onset" group was similar to that of the general population, while the proportion of predisposing heterodimers in patients diagnosed after 180 days of life was similar to that found in patients with typical type 1 DM. Accordingly, "early onset" children were less likely to have positive pancreatic autoantibodies than children with onset after 180 days (15.4% vs. 65.0%). Being small for gestational age at birth, a possible sign of impaired secretion and anabolic action of insulin, was more common in the "early onset" group. Three patients, who presented with DM within the first month of life, were small for date at birth, required continuous insulin therapy from the day of DM diagnosis, and were also affected by autoimmune enteropathy. Shortly before the above-mentioned study, mutations in FOXP3 had been identified as responsible for a syndromic autoimmune form of neonatal DM defined as IPEX syndrome (Immune dysregulation, Polyendocrinopathy, Enteropathy, X-linked syndrome) [16, 17]. IPEX was the only form of monogenic autoimmune neonatal DM for a long time and testing pancreatic autoimmunity in patients with DM onset within 6 months of life was not considered essential. More recently, mutations in four different autosomal genes have been identified in patients with neonatal DM characterized by positive pancreatic autoantibodies and autoimmune destruction of the pancreatic beta cell, in the context of an IPEX-like syndrome [18].

In *2004*, Gloyn et al. [19] hypothesized that activating mutations in the gene encoding potassium inwardly rectifying channel, subfamily J, member 11 (KCNJ11) cause neonatal DM, because it was already known that inactivating mutations in the same gene caused uncontrolled insulin secretion and congenital hyperinsulinism [20]. KCNJ11 gene encodes the pore-forming subunit (KIR6.2) of the ATP-sensitive potassium channel (KATP) in pancreatic beta cells. KIR6.2 forms a hetero-octameric complex with the sulfonylurea receptor subtype 1 (SUR1) encoded by the adenosine triphosphate (ATP)-binding cassette, subfamily C, member 8 (ABCC8) gene. Sulfonylureas bind to SUR1 and cause channel closure and insulin secretion. Six novel, heterozygous missense mutations were identified in 10 of the 29 analyzed patients. In 2 patients neonatal DM was familial, while 8 cases carried a new (non-inherited) mutation. In some patients neonatal DM was associated with severe developmental delay, muscle weakness, epilepsy, and mild dysmorphic features

(Developmental delay, Epilepsy, and Neonatal Diabetes: DEND syndrome). In *2006*, activating mutations in ABCC8 gene, encoding SUR1, were also identified in 9 patients with permanent or transient neonatal DM [21]. Patients with KCNJ11 or ABCC8 mutations were not able to secrete insulin in response to glucose or glucagon, but they secreted insulin in response to tolbutamide. This groundbreaking discovery opened the possibility to switch these children from subcutaneous insulin to oral sulfonylureas, with a remarkable improvement in blood glucose control and quality of life [22]. Initially, commercial brands of glibenclamide tablets were finely crushed into powder for infants and children who were too young to swallow tablets and/or required doses that were too low to be reliably obtained using the tablets. The powder obtained was resuspended in sterile water at a concentration of 5 mg/ml (or 0.25 mg/drop) and administered as an oral suspension in three daily doses [22]. More manageable pharmaceutical preparations have been recently proposed [23].

In *2007*, Stoy et al. [24] first reported that mutations in the promoter of the insulin gene (INS) can cause permanent neonatal DM. Since then, INS gene mutations have been identified not only in children affected by permanent neonatal diabetes, but also in patients with maturity-onset diabetes of the young (MODY), patients with autoantibody-negative type 1 DM, and early-onset type 2 DM [25].

It is now well established that most patients with DM onset within the first 6 months of life do not have autoimmune type 1 DM, but carry an aberration of chromosome 6 or a pathogenic mutation of a single gene. Most mutations are located in genes involved in pancreatic embryogenesis and lead to pancreas agenesis or hypoplasia (in some cases associated with major malformations in other organs), or beta cell dysfunction with impaired synthesis and secretion of insulin. Nevertheless, monogenic defects leading to early autoimmune aggression of different organs including the endocrine pancreas have been described. Consequently, neonatal DM is now clearly distinct from type 1 and type 2 DM.

In *2015*, the results of a comprehensive genomic testing in a series of 1020 patients with DM presenting before 6 months of age were published [26]. Causal mutations were found in 82% of the cases after Sanger sequencing, 6q24 methylation analysis, and targeted next-generation sequencing of all genes known as causative of neonatal DM. Mutations in the potassium channel genes (KCNJ11 and ABCC8) were the most common cause (38.2%) of neonatal DM but were identified less frequently in consanguineous families (12% in consanguineous families vs. 46% in non-consanguineous families). Mutations in the INS gene were found in 10% of patients from both non-consanguineous and consanguineous families. A homozygous mutation in EIF2AK3 gene responsible for Wolcott–Rallison syndrome, a rare autosomal recessive syndrome characterized by permanent neonatal DM, pancreas exocrine insufficiency, growth retardation with skeletal dysplasia, and severely impaired liver function [27], was the most common genetic cause in consanguineous families (24%). Overexpression of the imprinted region of chromosome 6q24, due to the duplication of 6q24 from either UPD or unbalanced duplication of the paternal chromosome 6, was found in 20% of patients with transient neonatal DM.

It is currently estimated that around 20% of neonatal DM cases still remain without a genetic diagnosis.

References

1. Besser RE, Flanagan SE, Mackay DG, Temple IK, Shepherd MH, Shields BM, et al. Prematurity and genetic testing for neonatal diabetes. Pediatrics. 2016;138(3). https://doi.org/10.1542/peds.2015-3926
2. Fösel S. Transient and permanent neonatal diabetes. Eur J Pediatr. 1995;154(12):944–8. https://doi.org/10.1007/BF01958635.
3. Joslin EP, Root HF, White P, Marble A. Treatment of diabetes mellitus, ed. 7, Philadelphia, Lea & Febiger, 1940, pp. 42, 48, 687, 692.
4. Rollo, cited by Magnano P. Ospedale maggiore. 1931;19:107.
5. Kitselle. Jhrb Kinderheilk. 1852;18:313.
6. Cuno F. Jb KinderheiLk. 1910;71:623.
7. Ramsey WR. Glycosuria of the newborn. treated with insulin. Trans Amer Pediat Soc. 1926;38:100–1.
8. Lawrence RD, McCance RA. Gangrene in an infant associated with temporary diabetes. Arch Dis Child. 1931;6(36):343–56. https://doi.org/10.1136/adc.6.36.343.
9. White P. Diabetes in childhood and adolescence, vol. 184. Philadelphia: Lea & Febiger; 1932. p. 859.
10. Lewis E, Eisenberg H. Diabetes mellitus neonatorum: report of a probable case. Am J Dis Child. 1935;49(2):408–10. https://doi.org/10.1001/archpedi.1935.01970020123012.
11. Limper MA, Miller AJ. Diabetes mellitus with extensive gangrene in early infancy. Am J Dis Child. 1935;50(5):1216–30. https://doi.org/10.1001/archpedi.1935.01970110124017.
12. Schwartzman J, Crusius ME, Beirne DP. Diabetes mellitus in infants under one year of age: report of a case and review of the literature. Am J Dis Child. 1947;74(5):587–606. https://doi.org/10.1001/archpedi.1947.02030010601004.
13. Hutchinson JH, Keay AJ, Kerr MM. Congenital temporary diabetes mellitus. Br Med J. 1962;2(5302):436–40. https://doi.org/10.1136/bmj.2.5302.436.
14. Temple IK, James RS, Crolla JA, Sitch FL, Jacobs PA, Howell WM, et al. An imprinted gene(s) for diabetes? Nat Genet. 1995;9(2):110–2. https://doi.org/10.1038/ng0295-110.
15. Iafusco D, Stazi MA, Cotichini R, Cotellessa M, Martinucci ME, Mazzella M, et al. Permanent diabetes mellitus in the first year of life. Diabetologia. 2002;45(6):798–804. https://doi.org/10.1007/s00125-002-0837-2
16. Wildin RS, Ramsdell F, Peake J, Faravelli F, Casanova JL, Buist N, et al. X-linked neonatal diabetes mellitus, enteropathy and endocrinopathy syndrome is the human equivalent of mouse scurfy. Nat Genet. 2001;27(1):18–20. https://doi.org/10.1038/83707.
17. Bennett CL, Christie J, Ramsdell F, Brunkow ME, Ferguson PJ, Whitesell L, et al. The immune dysregulation, polyendocrinopathy, enteropathy, X-linked syndrome (IPEX) is caused by mutations of FOXP3. Nat Genet. 2001;27(1):20–1. https://doi.org/10.1038/83713.
18. Johnson MB, Hattersley AT, Flanagan SE. Monogenic autoimmune diseases of the endocrine system. Lancet Diabetes Endocrinol. 2016;4(10):862–72. https://doi.org/10.1016/S2213-8587(16)30095-X.
19. Gloyn AL, Pearson ER, Antcliff JF, Proks P, Bruining GJ, Slingerland AS, et al. Activating mutations in the gene encoding the ATP-sensitive potassium-channel subunit Kir6.2 and permanent neonatal diabetes. N Engl J Med. 2004;350(18):1838–49. https://doi.org/10.1056/NEJMoa032922
20. Thomas P, Ye Y, Lightner E. Mutation of the pancreatic islet inward rectifier Kir6.2 also leads to familial persistent hyperinsulinemic hypoglycemia of infancy. Hum Mol Genet. 1996;5(11):1809–12. https://doi.org/10.1093/hmg/5.11.1809.
21. Babenko AP, Polak M, Cavé H, Busiah K, Czernichow P, Scharfmann R, et al. Activating mutations in the ABCC8 gene in neonatal diabetes mellitus. N Engl J Med. 2006;355(5):456–66. https://doi.org/10.1056/NEJMoa055068.
22. Tonini G, Bizzarri C, Bonfanti R, Vanelli M, Cerutti F, Faleschini E, et al. Sulfonylurea treatment outweighs insulin therapy in short-term metabolic control of patients with perma-

nent neonatal diabetes mellitus due to activating mutations of the KCNJ11 (KIR6.2) gene. Diabetologia. 2006;49(9):2210–3. https://doi.org/10.1007/s00125-006-0329-x.
23. Beltrand J, Baptiste A, Busiah K, Bouazza N, Godot C, Boucheron A, et al. Glibenclamide oral suspension: suitable and effective in patients with neonatal diabetes. Pediatr Diabetes. 2019;20(3):246–54. https://doi.org/10.1111/pedi.12823.
24. Støy J, Edghill EL, Flanagan SE, Ye H, Paz VP, Pluzhnikov A, et al. Insulin gene mutations as a cause of permanent neonatal diabetes. Proc Natl Acad Sci USA. 2007;104(38):15040–4. https://doi.org/10.1073/pnas.0707291104
25. Nishi M, Nanjo K. Insulin gene mutations and diabetes. J Diabetes Investig. 2011;2(2):92–100. https://doi.org/10.1111/j.2040-1124.2011.00100.x.
26. De Franco E, Flanagan SE, Houghton JA, Lango Allen H, Mackay DJ, Temple IK, et al. The effect of early, comprehensive genomic testing on clinical care in neonatal diabetes: an international cohort study. Lancet. 2015;386(9997):957–63. https://doi.org/10.1016/S0140-6736(15)60098-8.
27. Habeb AM, Flanagan SE, Deeb A, Al-Alwan I, Alawneh H, Balafrej AA, Mutair A, Hattersley AT, Hussain K, Ellard S. Permanent neonatal diabetes: different aetiology in Arabs compared to Europeans. Arch Dis Child. 2012 Aug;97(8):721–3. https://doi.org/10.1136/archdischild-2012-301744.

Chapter 2
Pathogenesis (of Neonatal Diabetes and Early Onset Diabetes)

Fabrizio Barbetti, Novella Rapini, and Stefano Cianfarani

2.1 Definition and Scope

Over the last 25 years, the concept of "neonatal diabetes mellitus" (NDM) has transitioned from a vague, indistinct entity [1] to a complex and well-defined array of conditions characterized by severe hyperglycemia presenting in the first 6 months of life, and beyond.

It is now well established that most of the NDM cases are associated with monoallelic or biallelic pathogenic variants of a single gene involved in the pancreatic β-cell function or with chromosomal aberrations of 6q24, as detailed in Chap. 4 (Classification of Neonatal and Early onset diabetes). Not surprisingly mechanism(s) of hyperglycemia of NDM depends on the gene-specific role in β-cell biology and on the nature of the genetic defect. Thus, NDM genes can be categorized into three broad functional areas that may occasionally overlap:

1. Genes of pancreas development and/or pancreatic islet/β-cell specification and/or maintenance of β-cell identity. Genes that regulate transcription of the insulin gene and/or of genes encoding for proteins involved in insulin secretion. This broad category included NDM caused by mutations in transcription factors.

Supplementary Information The online version contains supplementary material available at https://doi.org/10.1007/978-3-031-07008-2_2.

F. Barbetti (✉)
Monogenic Diabetes Clinic, Endocrinology and Diabetes Unit,
Bambino Gesù Children's Hospital, Rome, Italy
e-mail: Fabrizio.Barbetti@OPBG.net

N. Rapini · S. Cianfarani
Endocrinology and Diabetes Unit, Bambino Gesù Children's Hospital, Rome, Italy

I. Rabbone, D. Iafusco (eds.), *Neonatal and Early Onset Diabetes Mellitus*,
https://doi.org/10.1007/978-3-031-07008-2_2

2. Genes of unfolded protein response/endoplasmic reticulum stress (ER) regulation within the pancreatic β-cell. Insulin gene mutations as a trigger of sustained, unresolvable ER stress.
3. Genes of metabolic signaling of insulin secretion.

In addition, monogenic diabetes can originate from pathogenic variants in genes impacting immune system regulation, as beautifully described in the chapter on Classification of neonatal diabetes.

In this chapter, we will review in some detail the main three mechanisms of disease taking place in neonatal diabetes mellitus and childhood diabetes mellitus.

Genes of pancreas development and/or pancreatic islet/β-cell specification and/or maintenance of β-cell identity. Genes that regulate transcription of the insulin gene and/or of genes encoding for proteins involved in insulin secretion. Five examples.

PDX1/IPF1 A role for pancreatic development in Xenopus laevis of homeobox gene XIHBox8, the homologue of Pdx1 has been proposed in 1988, and Pdx1's crucial role in mice has been confirmed in 1994 [2] with the creation of an pancreatic mouse carrying a homozygous Pdx1 (then called IPF1) gene knock out [2]. Previously, the selective expression of Pdx1 in mice pancreatic β-cells and its role in the regulation of insulin gene transcription had been demonstrated [3]. The identification of a homozygous null variant of PDX1/IPF1 as the cause of pancreatic agenesis in men followed in 1997 [4], establishing a paradigm for the role of transcription factors in the pathogenesis of the permanent form of NDM, i.e., PNDM associated with pancreas exocrine deficiency. More recently, some hypomorphic PDX1 variants have been described in patients with PNDM without exocrine manifestations and normal pancreatic size [5, 6] or with head of the pancreas visible at ultrasound [5, 6]. Interestingly, pancreatic glucagon resulted in normal or increased in 2 patients suggesting that only β-cells were affected [5]. This different clinical presentation can be explained by the residual function of hypomorphic—missense—variants that are normally expressed, are normally targeted to the nucleus and have normal chromatin occupancy, but reduced transactivation of target gene promoters [5]. Of interest, human pluripotent stem cells (hPSC) modified by gene editing to bear a PDX1 homozygous mutation can proceed to the definitive endoderm stage but are unable to reach the pancreatic progenitor stage [7]. Recent studies on PDX1 target genes have revealed the changing role of this gene in cells at the pancreatic progenitor stage and in the mature β-cells (i.e., islets), where genes associated with insulin secretion, glucose sensing and β-cell identity (e.g., KCNJ11, NKX6.-1, and MAFA) prevail over genes important in pancreas development (GATA4, NEUROG3, HNF1A) [8]. These experiments have confirmed the crucial role of PDX1 in the "adult" β-cell where it acts together with other two transcription factors (TF), NEUROD1 and MAFA, in the regulation of basal and glucose-stimulated insulin gene expression/transcription [9]. In addition, PDX1 expression is essential to preserve β-cell identity [10]. Finally, PDX1 is crucial for β-cell survival during ER stress [11] acting in combination with two other transcription factors, ATF4 and ATF5 (Activating Transcription Factor 4 and 5) both involved in several cellular pathways including the unfolded protein response (UPR) and apoptosis.

Interestingly, heterozygous mutations of PDX1, NEUROD1, and MAFA can give rise to monogenic diabetes in adolescence/adulthood (Maturity Onset Diabetes of the Young; MODY) indicating that haploinsufficiency of these genes is sufficient to severely impair β-cell function. PDX1-MODY is considered rare, but recently new cases have been identified in young patients [12–14] often misdiagnosed with type 2 adolescent diabetes [15]. Interestingly, most pathogenic variants are frameshift mutations [13–15].

NEUROD1 Mice lacking NeuroD1 develop severe diabetes 2 days after birth because of the arrest of development of pancreatic islets, especially in the β-cell component [16]. NeuroD1 is present in most adult β-cells and plays a crucial role in the regulation of insulin gene transcription [17, 18] in a cooperative manner with PDX1 [19] and other transcription factors. Biallelic mutations of NEUROD1 cause syndromic neonatal diabetes (see chapter on neonatal diabetes classification) with no sign of exocrine deficiency, while heterozygous NEUROD1 pathogenic variants are associated with a rare form of MODY. Notably, most patients with NEUROD1-MODY are identified as young adults, and only a few during adolescence and childhood [18]. Pathogenic variants are loss-of-function frameshift mutations determining premature stop codons or missense mutations located within or in the proximities of the helix-loop-helix HLH) domain of NEUROD1 (such as Arg103Pro, Glu110Lys, or Arg111Leu) that impair NEUROD1 transactivation function. It is conceivable that in NEUROD1-MODY patients diabetes is induced by a combination of a reduced β-cell mass and impaired insulin gene transcription.

RFX6 Many experimental data support the role of RFX6 in endocrine pancreas development, maintenance of adult β-cell identity, and insulin secretion [20–22], and it is not surprising that loss-of-function (stop codon), heterozygous RFX6 variants have been associated with MODY phenotype [23–26]. In addition, RFX6 missense variants have been also associated with MODY in South-East Asians [27]. Thus, while RXF6 biallelic variants cause syndromic PNDM (see chapter on neonatal diabetes classification) RFX6 haploinsufficiency is associated with MODY that is probably caused by a combination of decreased β-cell number and abnormal β-cell function. Of note, RFX6-MODY onset seems to occur a little bit earlier than PDX1-MODY and NUROD1-MODY that share similar mechanism(s) of disease.

NEUROG3 NEUROG3, a helix-loop-helix (HLH) transcription factor, has a peculiar timing of expression in human fetal life, where appears at the early differentiation stage of the pancreas endocrine lineage, at 8 weeks post-conception (wpc) [28]. Thereafter NEUROG3 transient, single-wave expression peaks between 10 and 14 wpc when the endocrine commitment of pancreatic progenitor cells takes place [29]. Biallelic mutations of NEUROG3 determine diabetes with onset in the neonatal period and during infancy [30, 31] strongly supporting the notion that NEUROG3 is not dispensable for islet cell development [32]. However, recent findings on two patients with homozygous NEUROG3 frameshift mutations and diabetes onset in childhood have challenged this view [33], suggesting that a limited number of progenitors can be differentiated into β-cells even in the absence of functional NEUROG3. In contrast, all patients with biallelic NEUROG3 mutations show enteric anendocrinosis, that leads to malabsorptive diarrhea. The difference in sensitivity to NEUROG3 mutations between intestine and pancreatic β-cell seems to be linked to enhanced poor stability of mutated NEUROG3 protein in the intestine [34].

PTF1A With a combination of classic linkage studies and candidate gene(s) approach, mutations in the coding region of PTF1A completely disrupting its function have been linked to syndromic neonatal diabetes mellitus with cerebellar agenesis [35, 36]. PTF1A was selected among other genes because of its expression pattern in the pancreas and in the cerebellum. Of interest, mice lacking Ptf1a were shown to recapitulate the human phenotype [36] thus illustrating the role of this gene in pancreas development [37, 38]. More recently, a hypomorphic homozygous missense mutation and more importantly, recessive mutations in a distal PTF1A enhancer, have been associated with isolated pancreatic agenesis [39, 40]. The latter paper illustrated how either homozygous or compound heterozygous base substitutions or a large deletion (7.6 kb) of the entire PTF1A gene enhancer were responsible for isolated pancreatic agenesis in 10 different kindreds. Functional studies determined that the enhancer has lineage-specific activity in human pancreatic progenitor cells (derived from human embryonic stem cells, hESC) that directly interacts with PTF1A promoter. In addition, it has been shown that these mutations disrupt binding sites of FOXA2 and PDX1, which are essential for pancreatic development [40]. In contrast, hPSC lacking PTF1A could be differentiated in polyhormonal β-like cells [7]. Interestingly, PTF1A distal enhancer mutations are now recognized as the most frequent cause of isolated pancreatic agenesis [41].

Other transcription factors involved in pancreas organogenesis and function cause diabetes in the neonate and during infancy or even adulthood. More specifically biallelic mutations of GLIS3, MNX1, NKX2–2, and heterozygous pathogenic variants of GATA4, GATA6, and HNF1B have been associated with neonatal diabetes, with the latter three also causing diabetes in childhood, adolescence and in young adults [42]. Spontaneous heterozygous mutations of CNOT1, part of the Ccr4 not complex, which is important in the regulation of mRNA stability as well as for human embryonic stem cells self-renewal, cause a rare syndromic subtype of pancreatic agenesis and holoprosencephaly [43].

A recent addition (November 2021) to the list of syndromic PNDM genes is *ONECUT1* (also known as HNF6). Biallelic mutations of ONECUT1 give rise to PNDM/childhood diabetes characterized by hypoplastic pancreas and absent or small gallbladder [44]. Interestingly, a ONECUT1 spontaneous, heterozygous mutation has been also associated to diabetes with onset in adolescence [44], suggesting that *ONECUT1* could also represent a very rare cause of MODY. Of interest, studies performed in hESC during differentiation toward pancreatic β-cells showed that *ONECUT1* expression peaks at the pancreatic endoderm (PE) and pancreatic progenitor (PP) stages. In addition, *ONECUT1* binds to pancreas-specific enhancers and promoters at the PP stage indicating its important function in endocrine pancreas specification [45].

Genes of unfolded protein response/endoplasmic reticulum (ER) stress regulation within the pancreatic β-cell. Insulin gene mutations as a trigger of sustained, unresolvable ER stress. Three examples.

EIF2AK3 Biallelic mutations of *EIF2AK3* cause Wolcott-Rallison syndrome, characterized by neonatal/infancy onset diabetes, skeletal dysplasia, and liver dysfunction [46]. *EIF2AK3* encodes for eukaryotic translation initiation factor 2-α kinase 3 (also called PERK), a resident protein of the endoplasmic reticulum (ER) that is involved in the unfolded protein response (UPR). Mutations disrupting the kinase activity of PERK abolish the phosphorylation of translation initiation factor eIF2α that in turn becomes unable to reduce protein synthesis, a crucial function to avoid sustained ER stress. For many years Wolcott–Rallison syndrome has been considered the prototype of monogenic diabetes due to apoptosis of the β-cell triggered by unresolved ER stress [47]. More recently, however, this view has been challenged by experiments suggesting that the decreased β-cell mass induced by complete PERK deficiency is linked to reduced cell proliferation after birth, rather than ER stress-induced apoptosis [48]. Moreover, other mechanism(s) associated with proinsulin accumulation and regulation of PERK activity by calcium levels in the ER may impact β-cell function [48]. It has to be noted that all evidences have been obtained in animal (mouse) or cellular models. Thus, even if the two mechanisms of disease are not mutually exclusive, a more definitive word on this issue is expected to come from human iPSC experiments.

YIPF5 Recently a new gene, *YIPF5*, causing PNDM/infancy-onset diabetes and pronounced microcephaly, has been published [49]. Six living probands from five unrelated families were identified, with diabetes onset between 4 weeks and 15 months of age. Experiments conducted in patients-derived induced pluripotent stem cells carrying biallelic mutations of *YIPF5* demonstrated that loss of *YIPF5* function allows in vitro differentiation into β-cell-like cells that are, however, prone to surrender to ER stress-induced apoptosis, when compared with isogenic cells in which the genetic defect had been corrected by CRISPR. Data obtained in the human EndoC-βH1 β-cell line confirmed that insulin production and secretion are not affected by *YIPF5* silencing, that instead impacts two branches of integrated stress response (ISR) [50], i.e., PERK and ATF6, and sensitizes cells to ER stress-induced apoptosis. Additional experiments in β-cell-like cells derived from human embryonic stem cells with complete *YIPF5* deficiency showed dramatic retention of proinsulin in the ER with increased immunoreactivity against chaperon BiP, a marker of ER stress [49]. YIPF5 adds up to other genes that cause PNDM because of ISR mulfunction [50]. Of note, many genes implicated in ER stress diabetes in the neonatal/infancy period, such as *EIF2S3*, *IER3IP1*, *EIF2B1*, or in children/adolescents/young adults like *WFS1*, *WFS2* (*CISD*) *DNAJC3*, *PPP1R15B*, and *TRMT10A*, also cause syndromic diabetes with severe disturbances of nervous system, including microcephaly [51].

Insulin Insulin gene (*INS*) mutations represent the second cause of PNDM after *KCNJ11* in non-consanguineous families. First reports showed that many *INS*-PNDM pathogenic variants disrupt one of the three conserved disulfide bridges of the molecule or change the wild-type residue into supernumerary cysteine [52, 53] leading to insulin misfolding, trapping of insulin inside the β-cell and sustained, unresolvable ER stress [51]. However, heterozygous missense changes not involving cysteine may also elicit ER stress and β-cell apoptosis, causing PNDM or childhood (MODY) diabetes [54]. In general, it is assumed that heterozygous proinsulin variants with severely impaired folding cause permanent neonatal diabetes, while variants with less pronounced effects on foldability cause MODY [55]. Some variants, however, have been associated with both phenotypes. The inhibition on the transport of wild-type proinsulin brought about by mutated proinsulin is an additional mechanism of disease in *INS*-PNDM (and *INS*-MODY) [56]. This mechanism of disease is exemplified also by the finding that an INS intronic variant leading to mutant transcripts and (likely) translation of abnormal proinsulin are detected in familial PNDM/MODY [55, 56]. Of note, *INS* variants have been described in the early 1980 that can be secreted into the bloodstream causing mild diabetes in adults or even hypoglycemia [57, 58]. Recently, it has been hypothesized that for at least one of these variants, the Phe48Ser (previously known as PheB24Ser, a familial hyperinsulinemia mutation), may trigger proteotoxic misfolding [55].

Finally, exceedingly rare, recessive mutations in the coding region of *INS* gene or in its promoter may lead to neonatal diabetes (both permanent and transient) through a different mechanism, i.e., dramatically reduced or abolished insulin synthesis [59].

Genes of metabolic signaling of insulin secretion. Four examples.

SLC2A2 *SLC2A2* encodes for glucose transporter 2 (GLUT2) which is considered the likely "best pal" of glucokinase (hexokinase IV) to guarantee glucose sensing of pancreatic β-cells in humans. Complete Glut2 insufficiency (Glut2 −/− mouse) leads to hyperglycemia/hypoinsulinemia in the mouse with concurrent hyperglucagonemia and high levels of β-hydroxybutyric acid [60]. In contrast, homozygous *SLC2A2* mutations leading to GLUT2 lacking functional hexose transport activity are found in patients with Fanconi-Bickel syndrome, characterized by hepatomegaly, fasting hypoglycemia, tubular nephropathy, and rickets [61]. *SLC2A2*/GLUT2 is expressed in multiple human tissues/cells (pancreas, liver, kidney, intestine, and central nervous system) where it plays pleiotropic functions [10, 62]. The copresence and abundance of GLUT1 and GLUT3 in the human pancreatic β-cell raised the hypothesis that other glucose transporters could be involved in insulin secretion regulation in humans [63]. Therefore, the discovery that some patients with biallelic mutations of *SLC2A2* may present transient neonatal diabetes in addition to later presentation of classical features of Fanconi syndrome was interpreted as an important clue of the GLUT2 role in human insulin secretion [64]. Since the first report in 2012, additional cases of PNDM were associated with biallelic or even heterozygous *SLC2A2* pathogenic variants [65, 66]. Recently, a homozygous variant of uncertain significance has been also linked to diabetes in an adolescent with pancreatitis [67].

GCK The main kinetic properties of hexokinase IV, better known as glucokinase (GK) for its preferential use of glucose as substrate, are ideally suited to carry out its function of glucose sensor of the β-cell: an $S_{0.5}$ of circa 8 mmol/L (144 mg/dl) and the lack of inhibition of enzymatic activity by reaction product glucose-6-phosphate [68]. A strong support to this view was the discovery in 1992 that heterozygous loss-of-function mutations of the gene encoding glucokinase, *GCK*, give rise to the most frequent cause of autosomal dominant, mild, and non-progressive fasting hyperglycemia in childhood, i.e., GCK-MODY [69].

Mice completely lacking *Gck* (*Gck−/−*) die within 2–3 days from birth because of severe hypoinsulinemic hyperglycemia (neonatal diabetes) [70]. Similarly, humans with biallelic, loss-of-function mutations of *GCK* show non-syndromic, neonatal diabetes with onset within 1 week from birth (*GCK*/PNDM) [71]. These patients do not secrete insulin even in the presence of severe hyperglycemia (glucose levels higher than 500 mg/dl) [71]. Of interest, *Gck*-knockout mice can survive beyond 10 days of life when treated with glibenclamide [72]. In contrast, attempts to control glucose metabolism of patients with GCK-PNDM with sulfonylureas gave conflicting results from no response (Rabbone I, Cerutti F, Barbetti F unpublished results; [73]) to mild improvement [74, 75]. Though GCK is also expressed in liver [68], in the hypothalamus, and in specialized cells of intestine [76], no evident extrapancreatic features have been described in patients GCK-PNDM (OMIM # 606176) or GCK-MODY so far. Notably, activating *GCK* mutations, by setting β-cell sensing at a lower glucose level, cause hyperinsulinemic hypoglycemia.

KCNJ11/ABCC8 The very first report of ATP action on potassium channels of the rat pancreatic β-cell backs to 1984, when Cook and Hales described the K^+ channel-specific inhibition by ATP on the cytoplasmic side of cell membranes [77]. This result was interpreted as a possible direct link between intracellular glucose metabolism and cell membrane K^+ permeability [77]. Further evidence of the role of intracellular ATP and ATP to ADP ratio on insulin secretion emerged rapidly [78], and the cloning of the two subunits of ATP-dependent K^+ (K_{ATP}) channels paved the way for new research avenues [79, 80]. The discovery that biallelic, loss-of-function mutations of *ABCC8* (encoding for the regulatory subunit of K_{ATP} channels sulfonylurea receptor 1; SUR1), cause what was then defined as Persistent Hyperinsulinemic Hypoglycemia of Infancy (PHHI), reinforced the notion of the crucial role of K_{ATP} channels in β-cell function [81]. PHHI, a condition characterized by unregulated insulin secretion and severe hypoglycemia (currently known as Hyperinsulinemic Hypoglycemia; HH or Congenital Hyperinsulinemia; CHI) can be caused also by loss-of-function mutations of *KCNJ11* gene, encoding for Kir6.2, i.e., the pore-forming subunit of K_{ATP} channels [82, 83]. These results further validated the concept of K_{ATP} channels as the mechanism by which β-cells set their resting membrane potential and act as a master regulator of insulin secretion [84]. Of much interest, a transgenic mouse expressing β-cell K_{ATP} channels with reduced sensitivity to ATP inhibition showed neonatal, hypoinsulinemic diabetes with ketoacidosis [85] providing the clue for investigating humans with mirror phenotype of HH, i.e., NDM. The clinical prediction proved true with the identification of gain of function, heterozygous mutations of *KCNJ11* as a frequent cause of NDM (permanent and transient) [86]. Two years later also gain-of-function mutations of *ABCC8* were associated with NDM [87]. Transgenic mice with overactive K_{ATP} in the β-cells showed normal pancreatic islet morphology and size and apparently normal insulin content [85]. In other words, these mice were capable to synthesize insulin in normal amounts but were unable to secrete it. A proof-of-concept that also pancreatic β-cells of humans with K_{ATP}-NDM are viable has been obtained with the observation of long-term efficacy of sulfonylurea therapy in these patients [88, 89].

Calcium channels Voltage-gated Ca^{++} channels (Ca_v) are involved in insulin secretion and are a matter of intense basic research [90–93]. However, no Ca_v genetic variant has been associated with monogenic diabetes to date. Recently, two patients with Liang-Wang syndrome (LIWAS) have been described who presented, in addition to typical LIWAS features, neonatal diabetes mellitus [94, 95], LIWAS is caused by mutations in *KCNMA1* gene, that encodes for the Ca^{2+} and voltage-activated K^+ channel (BKC). Further research is needed to establish whether BKC plays a role in insulin secretion or the observation was merely coincidental.

References

1. Von Muhlendahl KE, Herkenhoff H. Long-term course of neonatal diabetes. N Engl J Med. 1995;333:704–8.
2. Jonsson J, Carlsson L, Edlund Y, Edlund H. Insulin-promoter-factor 1 is required for pancreas development in mice. Nature. 1994;371:606–9.
3. Ohlsson H, Karlsson K, Edlund T. IPF1, a homeodomain-containing transactivator of the insulin gene. EMBO J. 1993;12:4251–9.
4. Stoffers DA, Zinkin NT, Stanojevic V, Clarke WL, Habener JF. Pancreatic agenesis attributable to a single nucleotide deletion in the human IPF1 gene coding sequence. Nat Genet. 1997;15:106–10. https://doi.org/10.1038/ng0197-106.
5. Nicolino M, Claiborn KC, Senée V, Boland A, Stoffers DA, Julier C. A novel hypomorphic PDX1 mutation responsible for permanent neonatal diabetes with subclinical exocrine deficiency. Diabetes. 2010;59:733–40.
6. De Franco E, Shaw-Smith C, Flanagan SE, Edghill EL, Wolf J, Otte V, Ebinger F, Varthakavi P, Vasanthi T, Edvardsson S, Hatttersley ES. Biallelic PDX1 (insulin promoter factor 1) mutations causing neonatal diabetes without exocrine pancreatic insufficiency. Diabet Med. 2013;30:e197–200.
7. Zhu Z, Qing V, Lee K, Rosen BP, Gonzalez F, Soh C-L, Huangfu D. Genome editing of lineage determinants in human pluripotent stem cells reveal mechanisms of pancreatic development and diabetes. Cell Stem Cell. 2016;18:755–68.
8. Wang X, Sterr M, Burtscher I, Chen S, Hieronimus A, Machicao F, Staiger H, Häring HU, Lederer G, Meitinger T, Cernilogar FM, Schotta G, Irmler M, Beckers J, Hrabě de Angelis M, Ray M, Wright CVE, Bakhti M, Lickert H. Genome-wide analysis of PDX1 target genes in human pancreatic progenitors. Mol Metab. 2018;9:57–68.
9. Andrali SS, Samoley ML, Vanderford NL, Ozcan S. Glucose regulation of insulin gene expression in pancreatic β-cells. Biochem J. 2008;415:1–10.
10. Rutter GA, Pullen TJ, Hodson DJ, Martinez-Sanchez A. Pancreatic β-cell identity, glucose sensing and the control of insulin secretion. Biochem J. 2015;466:203–18.

11. Sachdeva MM, Claiborn KC, Khoo C, Yang J, Groff DN, Mirmira RG, Stoffers DA. Pdx1 (MODY4) regulates pancreatic beta cell susceptibility to ER stress. Proc Natl Acad Sci U S A. 2009;19:19090–5.
12. Miss AGM, Tarantino RM, da Fonseca ACP, de Souza RB, Soares CAPD, Cabello PH, Rodacki M, Zajdenverg L, Zembrzuski VM, Campos JM. PDX1-MODY: a rare missense mutation as a cause of monogenic diabetes. Eur J Med Genet. 2021;64:104194.
13. Al-Kandari H, Al-Abdulrazzaq D, Davidsson L, Nizam R, Jacob S, Melhem M, John SE, Al-Mulla F. Identification of maturity-onset-diabetes of the young (MODY) mutations in a country where diabetes is endemic. Sci Rep. 2021;11:16060.
14. Breidbart E, Deng L, Lanzano P, Fan X, Guo J, Leibel RL, LeDuc CA, Chung WK. Frequency and characterization of mutations in genes in a large cohort of patients referred to MODY registry. J Pediatr Endocrinol Metab. 2021;34:633–8.
15. Kleinberger JW, Copeland KC, Gandica RG, Haymond MW, Levitsky LL, Linder B, Shuldiner AR, Tollefsen S, White NH, Pollin TI. Monogenic diabetes in overweight and obese youth diagnosed with type 2 diabetes: the TODAY clinical trial. Genet Med. 2018;20:583–90.
16. Naya FJ, Huang HP, Qiu Y, Mutoh H, DeMayo FJ, Leiter AB, Tsai MJ. Diabetes, defective pancreatic morphogenesis, and abnormal enteroendocrine differentiation in BETA2/neuroD-deficient mice. Genes Dev. 1997;11:2323–34.
17. Sharma A, Moore M, Marcora E, Lee JE, Qiu Y, Samaras S, Stein R. The NeuroD1/BETA2 sequences essential for insulin gene transcription colocalize with those necessary for neurogenesis and p300/CREB binding protein binding. Mol Cell Biol. 1999;19:704–13.
18. Horikawa Y, Enya M. Genetic dissection and clinical features of MODY 6 (NEUROD1-MODY). Curr Diab Rep. 2019;19:12.
19. Glick E, Leshkowitz D, Walker MD. Transcription factor BETA2 acts cooperatively with E2A and PDX1 to activate the insulin gene promoter. J Biol Chem. 2000;275:2199–204.
20. Piccand J, Strasser P, Hodson DJ, Meunier A, Ye T, Keime C, Birling MC, Rutter GA, Gradwohl G. Rfx6 maintains the functional identity of adult pancreatic β cells. Cell Rep. 2014;9:2219–32.
21. Chandra V, Albagli-Curiel O, Hastoy B, Piccand J, Randriamampita C, Vaillant E, Cavé H, Busiah K, Froguel P, Vaxillaire M, Rorsman P, Polak M, Scharfmann R. RFX6 regulates insulin secretion by modulating Ca2+ homeostasis in human β cells. Cell Rep. 2014;9:2206–18.
22. Jennings RE, Scharfmann R, Staels W. Transcription factors that shape the mammalian pancreas. Diabetologia. 2020;63:1974–80.
23. Patel KA, Kettunen J, Laakso M, Stančáková A, Laver TW, Colclough K, Johnson MB, Abramowicz M, Groop L, Miettinen PJ, Shepherd MH, Flanagan SE, Ellard S, Inagaki N, Hattersley AT, Tuomi T, Cnop M, Weedon MN. Heterozygous RFX6 protein truncating variants are associated with MODY with reduced penetrance. Nat Commun. 2017;8:888.
24. Akiba K, Ushijima K, Fukami M, Hasegawa Y. A heterozygous protein-truncating RFX6 variant in a family with childhood-onset, pregnancy-associated and adult-onset diabetes. Diabet Med. 2020;37:1772–6.
25. Imaki S, Iizuka K, Horikawa Y, Yasuda M, Kubota S, Kato T, Liu Y, Takao K, Mizuno M, Hirota T, Suwa T, Hosomichi K, Tajima A, Fujiwara Y, Yamazaki Y, Kuwata H, Seino Y, Yabe D. A novel RFX6 heterozygous mutation (p.R652X) in maturity-onset diabetes mellitus: a case report. J Diabetes Investig. 2021;12:1914–8.
26. Tosur M, Soler-Alfonso C, Chan KM, Khayat MM, Jhangiani SN, Meng Q, Refaey A, Muzny D, Gibbs RA, Murdock DR, Posey JE, Balasubramanyam A, Redondo MJ, Sabo A. Exome sequencing in children with clinically suspected maturity-onset diabetes of the young. Pediatr Diabetes. 2021;22:960–8.
27. Mohan V, Radha V, Nguyen TT, Stawiski EW, Pahuja KB, Goldstein LD, Tom J, Anjana RM, Kong-Beltran M, Bhangale T, Jahnavi S, Chandni R, Gayathri V, George P, Zhang N, Murugan S, Phalke S, Chaudhuri S, Gupta R, Zhang J, Santhosh S, Stinson J, Modrusan Z, Ramprasad VL, Seshagiri S, Peterson AS. Comprehensive genomic analysis identifies pathogenic variants

in maturity-onset diabetes of the young (MODY) patients in South India. BMC Med Genet. 2018;19:22.

28. Jennings RE, Berry AA, Kirkwood-Wilson R, Hearn T, Salisbury RJ, Blaylock J, Piper Hanley K, Hanley NA. Development of the human pancreas from foregut to endocrine commitment. Diabetes. 2013;62:3514–22.
29. Salisbury RJ, Blaylock J, Berry AA, Jennings RE, De Krijger R, Piper Hanley K, Hanley NA. The window period of NEUROGENIN3 during human gestation. Islets. 2014;6:e954436.
30. Jensen JN, Rosenberg LC, Hecksher-Sørensen J, Serup P. Mutant neurogenin-3 in congenital mal absorptive diarrhea. N Engl J Med. 2007;356:1781–2.
31. Rubio-Cabezas O, Jensen JN, Hodgson MI, Codner E, Ellard S, Serup P, Hattersley AT. Permanent neonatal diabetes and enteric anendocrinosis associated with biallelic mutations in NEUROG3. Diabetes. 2011;60:1349–453.
32. Schreiber V, Mercier R, Jiménez S, Ye T, García-Sánchez E, Klein A, Meunier A, Ghimire S, Birck C, Jost B, de Lichtenberg KH, Honoré C, Serup P, Gradwohl G. Extensive NEUROG3 occupancy in the human pancreatic endocrine gene regulatory network. Mol Metab. 2021;53:101313.
33. Solorzano-Vargas RS, Bjerknes M, Wang J, Wu SV, Garcia-Careaga MG, Pitukcheewanont P, Cheng H, German MS, Georgia S, Martín MG. Null mutations of NEUROG3 are associated with delayed-onset diabetes mellitus. JCI Insight. 2020;5:e127657.
34. Zhang X, McGrath PS, Salomone J, Rahal M, McCauley HA, Schweitzer J, Kovall R, Gebelein B, Wells JM. A comprehensive structure-function study of neurogenin3 disease-causing alleles during human pancreas and intestinal organoid development. Dev Cell. 2019;50:367–80.
35. Sellick GS, Garret C, Houlston RS. A novel gene for neonatal diabetes maps to chromosome 10p12.1-p13. Diabetes. 2003;52:2636–8.
36. Sellick GS, Barker KT, Stolte-Dijkstra I, Fleischmann C, Cleman RJ, Garrett C, Gloyn AL, Edghill EL, Hattersley AT, Wellauer PK, Goodwin G, Houlson RS. Mutations in PTF1A cause pancreatic and cerebellar agenesis. Nat Genet. 2004;36:1301–5.
37. Kapp A, Knöfler M, Ledermann B, Bürki K, Berney C, Zoerkler N, Hagenbüchle O, Wellauer PK. The bHLH protein PTF1-p48 is essential for the formation of the exocrine and the correct spatial organization of the endocrine pancreas. Genes Dev. 1998;12:3752–63.
38. Kawaguchi Y, Cooper B, Gannon M, Ray M, MacDonald RJ, Wright CV. The role of the transcriptional regulator PTF1A in converting intestinal to pancreatic progenitor. Nat Genet. 2002;32:128–34.
39. Houghton JAL, Swift GH, Shaw-Smith C, Flanagan SE, de Franco E, Caswell R, Hussain K, Mohamed S, Addulrasoul M, Hattersley AT, MacDobnald RJ, Ellard S. Isolated pancreatic aplasia due to a hypomorphic PTF1A mutation. Diabetes. 2016;65:2810–5.
40. Weedon MN, Cebola I, Patch A-M, Flanagan SE, de Franco E, Caswell R, Rodriguez-Segui SA, Shaw-Smith C, Cho CH-H, Marsh P, Vallier L, Murray A, International Pancreatic Agenesis Consortium, Ellard S, Ferre J, Hattersley AT. Recessive mutations in a distal PTF1A enhancer cause isolated pancreatic agenesis. Nat Genet. 2014;46:61–4.
41. Demirbelek H, Cayir A, Flanagan SE, Yildirim R, Kor Y, Gurbuz F, Haliloglu B, Yildiz M, Baran RT, Akbas ED, Demiral M, Unal ER, Arslan G, Vuralli D, Buyukyilmaz G, Al-Khawaga S, Saeed A, Maadheed AM, Khalifa A, Onal H, Yuksel B, Ozbek MN, Bereket A, Hattersly AT, Hussain K, De Franco E. Clinical characteristics and long-term follow-up of patients with diabetes due to PTF1A enhancer mutations. J Clin Endocrinol Metab. 2020;105:1–9.
42. De Franco E. From biology to genes and back again: gene discovery for monogenic forms of beta-cell dysfunction in diabetes. J Mol Biol. 2020;432:1535–50.
43. De Franco E, Watson RA, Weninger WJ, Wong CC, Flanagan SE, Caswell R, Green A, Tudor C, Lelliott CJ, Geyer SH, Maurer-Gesek B, Reissig LF, Lango Allen H, Caliebe A, Siebert R, Holterhus PM, Deeb A, Prin F, Hilbrands R, Heimberg H, Ellard S, Hattersley AT, Barroso I. A specific CNOT1 mutation results in a novel syndrome of pancreatic agenesis and holoprosencephaly through impaired pancreatic and neurological development. Am J Hum Genet. 2019;104:985–9.

44. Philippi A, Heller S, Costa IG, Senée V, Breunig M, Li Z, Kwon G, Russell R, Illing A, Lin Q, Hohwieler M, Degavre A, Zalloua P, Liebau S, Schuster M, Krumm J, Zhang X, Geusz R, Benthuysen JR, Wang A, Chiou J, Gaulton K, Neubauer H, Simon E, Klein T, Wagner M, Nair G, Besse C, Dandine-Roulland C, Olaso R, Deleuze JF, Kuster B, Hebrok M, Seufferlein T, Sander M, Boehm BO, Oswald F, Nicolino M, Julier C, Kleger A. Mutations and variants of ONECUT1 in diabetes. Nat Med. 2021;27:1928–40.
45. Heller S, Li Z, Lin Q, Geusz R, Breunig M, Hohwieler M, Zhang X, Nair GG, Seufferlein T, Hebrok M, Sander M, Julier C, Kleger A, Costa IG. Transcriptional changes and the role of ONECUT1 in hPSC pancreatic differentiation. Commun Biol. 2021;4:1298.
46. Julier C, Nicolino M. Wolcott-Rallison syndrome. Orphanet J Rare Dis. 2010;5:29.
47. Harding HP, Ron D. Endoplasmic reticulum stress and the development of diabetes. Diabetes. 2002;51(Suppl. 3):S455–61.
48. Cavener DR, Gupta S, McGrath BC. PERK in β-cell biology and insulin biogenesis. Trends Endocrinol Metab. 2010;21:714–21.
49. De Franco E, Lytrivi M, Ibrahim H, Montaser H, Wakeling MN, Fantuzzi F, Patel K, Demarez C, Cai Y, Igoillo-Esteve M, Cosentino C, Lithovius V, Vihinen H, Jokitalo E, Laver TW, Johnson MB, Sawatani T, Shakeri H, Pachera N, Haliloglu B, Ozbek MN, Unal E, Yildirim R, Godbole T, Yildiz M, Aydin B, Bilheu A, Suzuki I, Flanagan SE, Vanderhaeghen P, Senée V, Julier C, Marchetti P, Eizirik DL, Ellard S, Saarimäki-Vire J, Otonkoski T, Cnop M, Hattersley AT. YIPF5 mutations cause neonatal diabetes and microcephaly through endoplasmic reticulum stress. J Clin Invest. 2020;130:6338–53.
50. Costa-Mattioli WP. The integrated stress response: from mechanism to disease. Science. 2020;368:eaat 5314.
51. Cnop M, Toivonen S, Igoillo-Esteve M, Salpea P. Endoplasmic reticulum stress and eIF2α phosphorylation: the Achilles heel of pancreatic β cells. Molec Metab. 2017;6:1024–39.
52. Støy J, Edghill EL, Flanagan SE, Ye H, Paz VP, Pluzhnikov A, Below JE, Hayes MG, Cox NJ, Lipkind GM, Lipton RB, Greeley SA, Patch AM, Ellard S, Steiner DF, Hattersley AT, Philipson LH, Bell GI, Neonatal Diabetes International Collaborative Group. Insulin gene mutations as a cause of permanent neonatal diabetes. Proc Natl Acad Sci U S A. 2007;104:15040–4.
53. Colombo C, Porzio O, Liu M, Massa O, Vasta M, Salardi S, Beccaria L, Monciotti C, Toni S, Pedersen O, Hansen T, Federici L, Pesavento R, Cadario F, Federici G, Ghirri P, Arvan P, Iafusco D, Barbetti F, the Early onset diabetes Study Group of the Italian Society of Pediatric Endocrinology and Diabetes (SIEDP). Seven mutations in the human insulin gene linked to permanent neonatal/infancy-onset diabetes mellitus. J Clin Invest. 2008;118:2148–56.
54. Liu M, Sun J, Cui J, Chen W, Guo H, Barbetti F, Arvan P. INS-gene mutations: from genetics and beta cell biology to clinical disease. Mol Aspect Med. 2015;42:3–18.
55. Dhayalan B, Chatterjee D, Chen Y-C, Weiss MA. Structural lessons from the mutant proinsulin syndrome. Front Endocrinol. 2021;12:754693.
56. Liu M, Haataja L, Wright J, Wickramasinghe NP, Hua QX, Phillips NF, Barbetti F, Weiss MA, Arvan P. Mutant INS-gene induced diabetes of youth: proinsulin cysteine residues impose dominant-negative inhibition on wild-type proinsulin transport. PLoS One 5:e13333.
57. Matsuno S, Furuta H, Kosaka K, Doi A, Yorifuji T, Fukuda T, Senmaru T, Uraki S, Matsutani N, Furuta M, Mishima H, Iwakura H, Nishi M, Yoshiura K, Fukui M, Akamizu T. Identification of a variant associated with early-onset diabetes in the intron of the insulin gene with exome sequencing. J Diabetes Invest. 2019;10:947–50.
58. Barbetti F, Raben N, Kadowaki T, Cama A, Accili D, Gabbay KH, Merenich JH, Taylor SI, Roth J. Two unrelated patients with familial hyperproinsulinemia due to a mutation substituting histidine for arginine at position 65 in the proinsulin molecule: identification of the mutation by direct sequencing of genomic deoxyribonucleic acid amplified by polymerase chain reaction. J Clin Endocrinol Metab. 1990;71:164–9.
59. Ma S, Viola R, Sui L, Cherubini V, Barbetti F, Egli D. β cell replacement after gene editing of a neonatal diabetes-causing mutation at the insulin locus. Stem Cell Reports. 2018;11:1407–15.

60. Thorens B. A gene knockout approach in mice to identify sensors controlling glucose homeostasis. Pflugers Arch. 2003;445:482–90.
61. Santer R, Schneppenheim R, Dombrowski A, Götze H, Steinmann SJ. Mutations in GLUT2, the gene for the liver-type glucose transporter, in patients with Fanconi-Bickel syndrome. Nat Genet. 1997;17:324–6.
62. Thorens B. GLUT2, glucose sensing and glucose homeostasis. Diabetologia. 2015;58:221–32.
63. Baroni MG, Sentinelli F, Lovari S, Massa O, Romeo S, Colombo C, di Mario U, Barbetti F. Single-strand conformation polymorphism analysis of the glucose transporter gene GLUT 1 in maturity onset diabetes of the young. J Molec Med-JMM. 2001;79:270–4.
64. Sansbury FH, Flanagan SE, Houghton JA, Shuixian Shen FL, Al-Senani AM, Habeb AM, Abdullah M, Kariminejad A, Ellard S, Hattersley AT. SLC2A2 mutations can cause neonatal diabetes, suggesting GLUT2 may have a role in human insulin secretion. Diabetologia. 2012;55:2381–5.
65. Al-Khawaga S, Mohammed I, Saraswathi S, Haris B, Hasnah R, Saeed A, Almabrazi H, Syed N, Jithesh P, El Awwa A, Khalifa A, AlKhalaf F, Petrovski G, Abdelalim EM, Hussain K. The clinical and genetic characteristics of permanent neonatal diabetes (PNDM) in the state of Qatar. Mol Genet Genomic Med. 2019;7:e00753.
66. Ibrahim MN, Laghari TM, Riaz M, Khoso Z, Khan YN, Yasir M, Hanif MI, Flanagan SE, De Franco E, Raza J. Monogenic diabetes in Pakistani infants and children: challenges in a resource poor country. J Pedaitr Endocrinol Metab. 2021;34:1095–193.
67. Cheon CK, Lee YJ, Yoo S, Lee JH, Lee JE, Kim HJ, Choi IJ, Choi Y, Lee S, Yoon JY. Delineation of the genetic and clinical spectrum, including candidate genes, of monogenic diabetes: a multicenter study in South Korea. J Pedaitr Endocrinol Metab. 2020;33:1539–50.
68. Matschinsky FM. Regulation of pancreatic β-cell glucokinase. From basics to therapeutics. Diabetes. 2002;51(Suppl. 3):S394–404.
69. Froguel P, Zouali H, Vionnet N, Velho G, Vaxillaire M, Sun F, Lesage S, Soffel M, Takeda J, Passa P, Permautt AM, Beckmann JS, Bell GI, Cohen D. Familial hyperglycemia due to mutations in glucokinase. Definition of a subtype of diabetes mellitus. N Engl J Med. 1993;328:697–702.
70. Grupe A, Hultgren B, Ryan A, Ma YH, Bauer M, Stewart TA. Transgenic knockouts reveal a critical requirement for pancreatic β cell glucokinase in maintaining glucose homeostasis. Cell. 1995;83:69–78.
71. Njolstad PR, Sovik O, Cuesta-Munoz A, Bjorkhaug L, Massa O, Barbetti F, Undlien D, Shiota C, Magnuson MA, Molven A, Matschinsky FM, Bell GI. Neonatal diabetes mellitus due to complete glucokinase deficiency. N Engl J Med. 2001;344:1588–92.
72. Terauchi Y, Sakura H, Yasuda K, Iwamoto K, Takahashi N, Ito K, Kasai H, Suzuki H, Ueda O, Kamada N, Jishge K, Komeda K, Noda M, Kanazawa Y, Taniguchi S, Miwa I, Akanuma Y, Kodama T, Yazaki Y, Kadowaki T. Pancreatic beta-cell-specific targeted disruption of glucokinase gene. Diabetes mellitus due to defective insulin secretion to glucose. J Biol Chem. 1995;270:30253–6.
73. Oriola J, Morteno F, Gutierrez-Nogués A, Leon S, Garcia-Herrero C-M, Vincent O, Navas M-A. Lack of glibenclamide response in a case of permanent neonatal diabetes caused by incomplete inactivation of glucokinase. JIMD Rep. 2015;20:21–6.
74. Turkkahraman D, Bircan I, Tribble ND, Akçurin S, Ellard S, Gloyn AL. Permanent neonatal diabetes mellitus caused by a novel homozygous (T168A) glucokinase (GCK) mutation: initial response to oral sulphonylurea therapy. J Pediatr. 2008;153:122–6.
75. Bennet K, James C, Al-Shaik H, Sinani A, Hussain K. Four novel cases of permanent neonatal diabetes mellitus caused by homozygous mutations in the glucokinase gene. Pediatr Diabetes. 2011;12:192–6.
76. Seino Y, Maekawa R, Ogata H, Hayashi Y. Carbohydrate-induced secretion of the glucose-dependent insulinotropic polypeptide and glucagon-like peptide-1. J Diabetes Invest. 2016;7:27–32.

77. Cook DL, Hales CN. Intracellular ATP directly blocks K+ channels in pancreatic B-cells. Nature. 1984;311:271–3.
78. Ashcroft FM, Rorsman P. Electrophysiology of the pancreatic β-cell. Prog Biophys Molec Biol. 1989;54:87–143.
79. Ho K, Nichols CG, Lederer WJ, Lytton J, Vassilev PM, Kanazirska MV, Hebert SC. Cloning and expression of an inwardly rectifying ATP-regulated potassium channel. Nature. 1993;362:31–8.
80. Aguilar-Bryan L, Nichols CG, Wechsler SW, Clement JP 4th, Boyd AE 3rd, González G, Herrera-Sosa H, Nguy K, Bryan J, Nelson DA. Cloning of the beta cell high-affinity sulfonylurea receptor: a regulator of insulin secretion. Science. 1995;268:423–6.
81. Thomas PM, Cote GJ, Wohllk N, Haddad B, Mathew PM, Rabl W, Aguilar-Bryan L, Gagel RF, Bryan J. Mutations in the sulfonylurea receptor gene in familial persistent hyperinsulinemic hypoglycemia of infancy. Science. 1995;268:426–9.
82. Thomas P, Ye Y, Lightner E. Mutation of the pancreatic islet inward rectifier Kir6.2 also leads to familial persistent hyperinsulinemic hypoglycemia of infancy. Hum Molec Genet. 1996;5:1809–12.
83. Loechner KJ, Akrouh A, Kurata HT, Dionisi-Vici C, Maiorana A, Pizzoferro M, Rufini V, Ville de Goyet J, Colombo C, Barbetti F, Koster JC, Nichols CG. Congenital hyperinsulinism and glucose hypersensitivity in homozygous and heterozygous carriers of Kir6.2 (KCNJ11) mutation V290M mutation. K_{ATP} channel inactivation mechanism and clinical management. Diabetes. 2011;60:209–17.
84. Aguilar-Bryan L, Bryan J. Molecular biology of adenosine triphosphate-sensitive potassium channels. Endocr Rev. 1999;20:101–35.
85. Koster JC, Marshall BA, Ensor N, Corbett JA, Nichols CG. Targeted overactivity of beta cell K(ATP) channels induces profound neonatal diabetes. Cell. 2000;100:645–54.
86. Gloyn AL, Pearson ER, Antcliff JF, Proks P, Bruining GJ, Slingerland AS, Howard N, Srinivasan S, Silva JM, Molnes J, Edghill EL, Frayling TM, Temple IK, Mackay D, Shield JP, Sumnik Z, van Rhijn A, Wales JK, Clark P, Gorman S, Aisenberg J, Ellard S, Njølstad PR, Ashcroft FM, Hattersley AT. Activating mutations in the gene encoding the ATP-sensitive potassium-channel subunit Kir6.2 and permanent neonatal diabetes. N Engl J Med. 2004;350:1838–49.
87. Babenko AP, Polak M, Cavé H, Busiah K, Czernichow P, Scharfmann R, Bryan J, Aguilar-Bryan L, Vaxillaire M, Froguel P. Activating mutations in the ABCC8 gene in neonatal diabetes mellitus. N Engl J Med. 2006;355:456–66.
88. Bowman P, Sulen A, Barbetti F, Beltrand J, Svalastoga P, Codner E, Tessmann EH, Juliusson P, Skrivarhaug S, Pearson ER, Flanagan SE, Babiker T, Thomas NJ, Shepherd MH, Ellard S, Klimes I, Szopa M, Polak M, Iafusco D, Hattersley AT, Njolstad PR for the Neonatal Diabetes International Collaborative Group. Effectiveness and safety of long-term treatment with sulfonylureas in patients with neonatal diabetes due to KCNJ11 mutations: an international cohort study. Lancet Diabetes Endocrinol. 2018;6:637–46.
89. Bowman P, Mathews F, Barbetti F, Sheperd MH, Sanchez J, Piccini B, Beltrand J, Letourneau-Freiberg LR, Polak M, Greeley SAW, Rawlins E, Babiker T, Thomas MJ, De Franco E, Ellard S, Flanagan SE, Hattersley AT. Long-term follow-up of glycemic and neurological outcomes in an international series of patients with sulfonylurea-treated ABCC8 permanent neonatal diabetes. Diabetes Care. 2021;44:35–42.
90. Yang S-N, Berggren P-O. The role of voltage-gated calcium channels in pancreatic b-cell physiology and pathophysiology. Endocr Rev. 2006;27:621–76.
91. García-Delgado N, Velasco M, Sánchez-Soto C, Díaz-García CM, Hiriart M. Calcium channels in postnatal development of rat pancreatic beta cells and their role in insulin secretion. Front Endocrinol. 2018;9:40.
92. González-Ramírez R, Felix R. Transcriptional regulation of voltage-gated Ca^{2+} channels. Acta Physiol. 2018;222(1)

93. Yu J, Shi Y, Zhao K, Yang G, Yu L, Li Y, Andersson EM, Ämmälä C, Yang SN, Berggren PO. Enhanced expression of β cell Ca_V 3.1 channels impairs insulin release and glucose homeostasis. Proc Natl Acad Sci. 2020;117:448–53.
94. Liang L, Li X, Moutton S, Schrier Vergano SA, et al. De novo loss-of-function KCNMA1 variants are associated with a new multiple malformation syndrome and a broad spectrum of developmental and neurological phenotypes. Hum Mol Genet. 2019;28:L2937–51.
95. Mameli C, Cazzola R, Spaccini L, et al. Neonatal diabetes in patients affected by Liang-Wang syndrome carrying KCNMA1 variant p.(Gly375Arg) suggest a potential role of Ca^{2+} and voltage-activated K^+ channel activity in human insulin secretion. Curr Issues Mol Biol. 2021;43:1036–42.

Chapter 3
Epidemiology

Maurizio Delvecchio, Federica Ortolani, Alessandra Rutigliano, Marcella Vendemiale, and Elvira Piccinno

3.1 Background

Neonatal diabetes mellitus (NDM) is considered a rare disease coded as ORPHA:224 in the Orphanet database. The incidence is estimated to be approximately 1:20,000–350,000 live births, but it is more frequent (up to 1:21,000) in those Countries where consanguinity has a high rate [1, 2]. It can be classified as transient (TNDM) and permanent (PNDM), and in a minority of cases it is associated with other syndromes. The clinical manifestations are clear and its definition has been updated over the last two decades, affecting the estimation of incidence. It is unlikely that it could not be diagnosed, but it should be taken into consideration that neonatal hyperglycemia may occur in several conditions without being a sign of neonatal diabetes. In this chapter, we describe the epidemiology of neonatal diabetes mellitus in different Countries, aiming to point out the differences in incidence and genetic cause.

In the first part, we discuss in brief about neonatal hyperglycemia, which is strikingly more frequent than neonatal diabetes and should be confused with it. In the second part, we provide an overview of historical data about the incidence and frequency of neonatal diabetes mellitus and early onset diabetes. In the third part, we present data for geographical areas of the World.

Supplementary Information The online version contains supplementary material available at https://doi.org/10.1007/978-3-031-07008-2_3.

M. Delvecchio (✉) · F. Ortolani · A. Rutigliano · E. Piccinno
Metabolic disorders and Genetic Disease Unit, "Giovanni XXIII" Children's hospital, Bari, Italy

M. Vendemiale
Psychological Departmental Unit, "Giovanni XXIII" Children's hospital, Bari, Italy

I. Rabbone, D. Iafusco (eds.), *Neonatal and Early Onset Diabetes Mellitus*, https://doi.org/10.1007/978-3-031-07008-2_3

3.2 Neonatal Hyperglycemia

The definition of neonatal hyperglycemia is still under debate. The most common ones are:

- Blood glucose >120–125 mg/dL or plasma glucose >145–150 mg/dL, irrespective of gestational or postnatal age or weight.
- Blood glucose >125 mg/dL in term and >150 mg/dL in preterm infants.
- Blood glucose >215 mg/dL at any time.

The most important risk factors for neonatal hyperglycemia are gestational age < 37 weeks, postnatal age < 72 h, birthweight <2500 g, hypoxia, infection, use of inotropes, lipid infusion, respiratory distress syndrome, sepsis, and obviously high glucose infusion rate. Hyperglycemia causes hyperosmolality with subsequent osmotic diuresis and dehydration. It is more common during the first week after birth, and most infants are asymptomatic or present signs of an underlying disorder (sepsis or others). The disappearance after the first week of life is the most important point to make a differential diagnosis with neonatal diabetes.

It is estimated that hyperglycemia occurs in less than 5% of full-term infants, in 65–70% of infants weighing 1000–1500 g, in about 70% of infants weighing <1000 g, and in 80% of infants weighing <750 g. In these situations, different mechanisms interplay accounting for increase in blood glucose: immaturity or defective glucoregulatory hormone control, poor insulin response, peripheral insulin resistance, inability to suppress glucose production, and glucose intolerance. In these cases, the treatment is to treat the underlying cause of hyperglycemia and/or stop medications that may cause hyperglycemia. Persistent hyperglycemia, overall in the case of parenteral nutrition, may require treatment with insulin [3].

3.3 Neonatal Diabetes Mellitus: General Overview

Neonatal diabetes is a monogenic form of diabetes that occurs within the first 6 months of life. The work-up of the diagnosis may affect the estimation of the incidence. Neonatal diabetes could be mistaken for neonatal hyperglycemia or even type 1 diabetes (most in the past). Actually, a proper differential diagnosis is based on some important key points that can drive the choice of running or not genetic testing. First, type 1 diabetes onset before the age of 6 months of life is extremely rare. Second, the presence of autoantibodies against β-cell antigens is the hallmark of type 1 diabetes but they can be found, although occasionally, in neonatal diabetes. Third, neonatal diabetes is usually defined by "a diabetes duration of at least 2 weeks" as an inclusion criterion, in order to distinguish it from occasional, short-lived neonatal hyperglycemia [4, 5].

Some cases of neonatal diabetes can be diagnosed later than 6 months of age, up to 12 months. However, in this age range most of these patients have type 1 diabetes and not monogenic diabetes. In addition, in the definition of aetiology in infants with diabetes, it is well acknowledged that autoantibodies against β-cell antigens may be found in patients carrying mutations in genes related to immune function (LRBA, FOXP3, or STAT3) but not type 1 diabetes mellitus [6]. These patients usually feature other immunological disorders and diabetes can occur before or later than other clinical features, but it is important in the diagnosis of neonatal diabetes or so-called early onset diabetes. In patients with permanent neonatal diabetes, the cause can be undiagnosed in up to 20% of them, while in patients with the transient form, genetic aetiology is usually found. Till date, more than 30 genes responsible for neonatal diabetes have been identified [7, 8].

The prevalence of the transient and permanent form is similar in most Western Countries, with less than 10% of infants with neonatal diabetes carrying a mutation in one of those genes responsible for syndromic diabetes. On the other hand, in those Countries where neonatal diabetes mellitus seems to be more prevalent, the transient form is less frequent. The most prevalent genetic defect in the permanent subtype is in imprinted genes or methylation defect in the chromosome 6q24 region, which accounts for up to 75% of all these cases. The remaining infants with transient neonatal diabetes carry a gene defect in any of the gene encodings for K-ATP channel subunits. More rarely, INS gene mutations may be found. In the permanent subtype, the most frequently mutated genes are those encoding for the K-ATP channel subunits (*KCNJ11* and *ABCC8*) and *INS*. Table 3.1 shows the distribution of the genetic causes of neonatal diabetes.

There are no comprehensive reviews on this topic in literature, but a protocol for a systematic review and meta-analysis to determine incidence, prevalence, and genetic cause of neonatal diabetes has been recently published [9]. The only systematic review about neonatal diabetes incidence and prevalence was run by Saraswathi et al. [10] and aimed to report on data from the Middle-East Region, where the rate of consanguinity is high leading to a higher incidence of neonatal diabetes mellitus, mostly due to homozygous mutations.

Table 3.1 Distribution of the genetic causes of neonatal diabetes

Permanent neonatal diabetes mellitus (45–55%)	Transient neonatal diabetes mellitus (35–45%)	Neonatal diabetes mellitus associated to rare syndrome (about 10%)
40–60% *KCNJ11* mutations 25–35% *INS* mutations 10–20% *ABCC8* mutations Other genes mutations	60–80% 6q24 abnormalities 10–20% *ABCC8* mutations 5–15% *KCNJ11* mutations Other genes mutations	*EIF2AK3* (most frequent), *FOXP3*, *GLIS3*, *PTF1A*, *RFX6*, *NEUROG3*, *GATA6*, *GATA 4*

Permanent and transient neonatal diabetes mellitus are more frequent in Countries where consanguinity is uncommon, while neonatal diabetes mellitus associated to rare syndrome is more frequent in Countries where consanguinity is common

3.4 Prevalence and Incidence

One of the first reports about the prevalence of diabetes in infants was performed by Imerslud when neonatal diabetes and early onset diabetes had not yet been distinguished. In 1959, he reported 118 patients with diabetes onset before the age of 2 years (only 13 before the age of 1 year, 0.34% of the study cohort) among 3847 patients with juvenile diabetes followed up at the Joslin Diabetes Centre in Boston between 1922 and 1956 [11]. Few decades later, 51 patients (1.08%) with onset in the first year of life were reported among 4702 children diagnosed with diabetes between 1983 and 1998 in Sweden. Approximately, we can say that authors before the 1990s show that 0.5% of patients with diabetes are diagnosed before 1 year of age [12].

The incidence of neonatal diabetes can be calculated from the number of cases and the annual birth rate of that area. Actually, it could be underestimated because not all cases are referred because of death or lack of referral, but in any way, it will reflect the minimum incidence and it is a reliable parameter.

In 1980s, an age-specific incidence of 6.2/100,000 per year was calculated for the patients treated at Oxford children's diabetic clinic for the age group 0–2 years [13]. Few years later, a higher incidence was reported in the same age group in a Norwegian cohort (10.9/100,000), higher than in Italian (1.7/100,000) and German reports (1.43–1.96/100,000) [14, 15]. However, these papers do not report neonatal diabetes and do not distinguish between the onset in the first and in the second year of life, when onset is considerably increased.

A report about NDM published in the mid-90s [12] reviewed 139 cases of neonatal diabetes. The authors showed that only 65 of them presented transient and 29 permanent diabetes, even if the differentiation remained doubtful because of the short follow-up period. In the same year, von Muhlendahl and Herkenkoff [4] recruited data from literature and from 230 pediatric Department and clinics from former West Germany and described 47 patients with neonatal diabetes, defined as onset during the first month of life and insulin requirement for more than 2 weeks. In addition, they recruited 10 patients with diabetes onset in the second or third month of life. They concluded that 26 (45.6%) of the 57 infants had permanent diabetes and the other ones had the transient subtype (54.4%), which relapsed between 7 and 20 years of age in 13 of 31 (41.9%). The overall incidence was 1 in 500,000 neonates.

More recently, data from a very large international database including more than 28,000 patients (diabetes onset <20 years) from 37 European centers and 11 non-European centers reported 54 patients (0.2% of the cohort) with neonatal diabetes in February 2016 [16].

The minimal annual incidence rate increased over time. Interesting data from a single referral center about patients from the UK, the Netherlands, and Poland shows that the minimum observed incidence ranged from <0.5 cases per million (period 1950–1970) to 1.9–3.8 cases per million live births (1985–2005) [17]. The increase can be only apparent because it is estimated by number of referrals and thus different explanations could account for this. First of all, increase in survival rate due to improvement in clinical care over time. Second, genetic facilities have increased over time and in particular during the last 30 years. Third, it is likely that the referral rate has increased over time because of the increased awareness about genetic mechanisms in neonatal diabetes.

The genetic causes of neonatal diabetes present some differences among the different areas of the world. Since the first time of gene sequencing, it is clear that de novo *KCNJ11* and *ABCC8* mutations are the most frequent causes of permanent neonatal diabetes at least in patients of European and Japanese origin, and 6q24 abnormalities are the most frequent ones in infants with transient neonatal diabetes. A different picture comes from the Countries where the rate of consanguinity is high, overall from the Middle-East, where homozygous mutations and syndromic diabetes are the most frequent cause of neonatal diabetes. Wolcot-Rallison syndrome is the most frequent cause of permanent neonatal diabetes in Arab patients, due to the high rate of consanguinity. However, in this society mutations in genes, which encode for K-ATP channels subunits are the most frequent cause of isolated neonatal diabetes.

Data from the French Neonatal Diabetes Mellitus Study Group on 174 unrelated patients with diabetes onset before 1 year of age, normal pancreas morphology, and recruited between 1995 and 2010 from 20 Countries reported that 27% of them did not present any mutation in the investigated gene. On the other hand, 23% of the patients presented 6p24 abnormalities, 7.5% an INS gene mutation, and 42.5% a K-ATP channel gene mutation (43 of 174, 34%, with a *KCNJ11* mutation, and 31 of 174, 24%, a *ABCC8* mutation). Four patients (5%) out of 79 presented DEND, and 13 (16%) intermediate DEND [18].

In the following section, we present available epidemiological from different Countries according to the Continents. Figure 3.1 displays the incidence in each Country (Table 3.1).

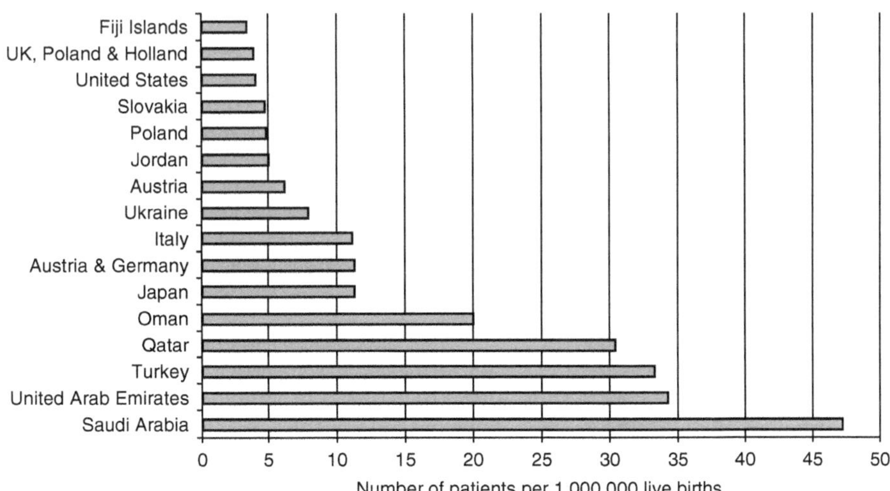

Fig. 3.1 Incidence of neonatal diabetes mellitus

3.5 Europe

3.5.1 Poland

The first observational study, which aimed to assess the prevalence of different subtypes of childhood diabetes, comes back to the period January 2005–December 2011. A prevalence of neonatal diabetes due to mutations in ABCC8 and KCNJ11 of 1/300,000–400,000 children is described [19]. A more comprehensive study, which evaluated the 11-year period from January 2005 to December 2015, recruited 788 probands under the age of 19 years and 813 family members with suspected monogenic diabetes [20]. The pediatric population in the areas overseen by the Centres involved in the study represented above the 40% of the Polish children. All of them underwent genetic testing for the most frequent causes of monogenic diabetes (*GCK*, *HNF1A*, *HNF1B*, *INS*, *KCNJ11*, *ABCC8*, *GATA6*, *GLIS3*, and *FOXP3*) with the following results: 322 (40.9%) of the 788 probands and 386 (47.5%) of 813 family members tested positive. The patients with permanent neonatal diabetes were 35 (10.9%) among the 322 probands, and 19 (4.9%) among the 386 family members. No patients were diagnosed with transient neonatal diabetes, and overall 31 (57.4%) of 54 patients carried a *KCNJ11* mutation. The other mutated genes were INS (11 patients, 20.4%), ABCC8 (6 patients, 11.1%), GCK (4 patients, 7.4%), GATA6 (2 patients, 3.7%), and FOXP3 (1 patient, 1.8%). The incidence of permanent neonatal diabetes was 0.48/100,000 children.

3.5.2 Germany and Austria

During the 18 years,1989–2007, 10 patients with neonatal diabetes were born in Austria. TNDM appears to be more frequent (70%) than PNDM (30%). However, a genetic diagnosis was confirmed only in 3 of 7 patients with TNDM and in 1 of 3 patients with PNDM. The overall estimated incidence was 1 in 160,949 live births (TNDM 1 in 229,928 live births and PNDM 1 in 536,499 live births). More recent epidemiological data are available from the Diabetes-Patienten-Verlaufsdokumentation, which is a large database including patients with diabetes onset before the age of 18 years from 229 Centers in Austria and Germany. The analysis of data entered by 2008 (more than 51,000 patients) showed that 90 patients presented diabetes mellitus onset before the age of 6 months. Interestingly, 7 patients out of 90 presented anti-β cells autoantibodies and were classified as type 1 diabetes and thus they were not considered for genetic analysis. The most frequently mutated gene was *KCNJ11* (10 patients), followed by *ABCC8* (7 patients). The presence of autoantibodies in so young patients does not rule out the diagnosis of monogenic diabetes, for instance, due to mutations in genes of autoimmunity (FOXP3, IL2RA, LRBA). The frequency of newly diagnosed DM in the period 2003–2007 was estimated at about 1 in 89,000 live births [21, 22].

3.5.3 *Italy*

Italian authors report a minimal incidence of neonatal diabetes mellitus of 1 in 90,000 live births in the 6-year period, 2005–2010 [23]. They recruited 27 patients with diabetes onset within the first 6 months of life, 16 with PNDM (59%) and 11 with TNDM (41%) that were screened for mutations in 3 genes (*KCNJ11*, *ABCC8*, and *INS*) and for 6q24 abnormalities. The most frequently mutated genes in PNDM were *KCNJ11* (7 in 16 patients, 43.7%) and *INS* (4 in 16 patients, 25%). Among the 11 patients with TNDM, the authors detected mutations of *KCNJ11* in 3 (27.3%), *ABCC8* in 3 (27.3%), and UDP in 1 patient. Five patients with PNDM and four patients with TNDM remained without a genetic diagnosis. Further data [24] showed that the incidence of PNDM was 1 in 210,287 live births (if onset occurs within the first 6 months of life) and 1 in 473,146 live births (if onset occurs within the first 6 weeks of life, previous definition of neonatal diabetes) in the period 1995–2009. Overall, the reports show that the most frequently mutated gene in Italian patients is *KCNJ11*, both in the case of transient and permanent neonatal diabetes. The prevalence of NDM is 0.6% among patients diagnosed with diabetes mellitus <18 years in the 6-year period 2007–2012 [25].

3.5.4 *Slovakia*

The incidence is estimated to be 1 in 215,417 live births in the period 1981–2004. Eight patients were born in that period, all of them with PNDM. A mutation in one of the genes related to NDM was found in 6 of them (one patient died without performing genetic testing and another one remained with unknown aetiology), with 4 of the 8 patients carrying a KCNJ11 gene mutation [26].

3.5.5 *Ukraine*

Epidemiological data are available from the Ukrainian Pediatric Diabetes Register between January 2012 and December 2014. Twelve cases with diabetes onset within 6 months of life were observed over 1,516,760 live births (incidence 1 in 126,397 live births). The authors found 46 patients with diabetes onset between 6 and 9 months of age reported in the database, with 24 of them with diabetes onset within the first 6 months of life. Forty-two patients underwent genetic testing and the detection rate was 86.4% (only 22 patients available for genetic testing), with *KCNJ11* mutations representing the most frequent cause (7 of 22), followed by *ABCC8* (4 patients for each). Four patients (of 20 available patients) with diagnosis later than 6 months of age carried a mutation in *INS* (3 patients) and *KCNJ11* (1 patient) [27].

3.6 Asia

3.6.1 China

Permanent neonatal diabetes is more frequent than the transient form in the Chinese population. In their report, Cao et al. [28] reported on 25 patients born between 2001 and 2013 at the Children's Hospitals in Beijing, Zhengzhou, and Shanxi. All of them had diabetes onset before the age of 6 months. Seven patients (28%) presented complete remission and were classified as transient, while 18 (72%) patients had permanent neonatal diabetes. Twelve mutations (66.6%) were identified among the 18 patients with PNDM (5 *KCNJ11*, 3 *EIF2AK3*, 1 *ABCC8*, 1 *INS*, 1 *GLIS3*, 1 *SLC19A2*). In the TNDM, three patients (42.8%) presented a mutation (2 cases in *ABCC* and 1 case with UPD6).

3.6.2 Japan

Few reports are available about the incidence of NDM in the Japanese population. A nationwide investigation carried out through a questionnaire involving nearly 1000 Pediatric and/or Neonatology Units (response rate 80%) showed an incidence of 1 in 89,000 newborns in the period 2007–2009. This incidence was higher than previously thought in this Country and similar to what was reported in some European Countries [29]. Transient and permanent neonatal diabetes appear to have a similar rate. 6q24 abnormalities are the most frequent aetiology in patients with NDM, while mutations in KCNJ11 gene are the most frequent cause of PNDM [30].

3.7 South Pacific

3.7.1 Fiji

Forty patients with diabetes onset <15 years of age were reported from 2001 to 2012, with a global incidence of 1.4 in 100,000 live births. Only one patient presented neonatal diabetes, with an estimated incidence of 1 in 300,000 live births [31].

3.8 Middle-East

3.8.1 Oman

In 1990s, the incidence of NDM (considered as hyperglycemia onset within the first month of life) was estimated to range from 1.8 to 2.2/100,000 live births, respectively, a figure nearly 5 time of what currently reported worldwide. The prevalence of PNDM was 2.4 per 100,000 children below 5 years of age, which was about 40% of all patients with diabetes mellitus. The high incidence is related to the rate of consanguineous marriage, which is more than half of all marriages. Familiar history showed consanguinity in all the cases of NDM born in that period [32].

A more recent report collected data about the patients born from 2007 to 2015. A genetic abnormality was detected in 15 of 24 patients, and homozygous mutation in GCK gene was the most frequent cause (7 patients in 15), unlike Western populations [33]. Again, this figure reflects the degree of consanguinity that is a traditional practice in the Middle East area.

3.8.2 Jordan

The reported incidence of PNDM is 1 in 203,221 live births in the period 2006–2012. A genetic cause was detected in 60% of the patients, in whom KCNJ11 gene mutations were the most frequent cause (50%). *EIF2AK3* mutations accounted for 20% of all cases with PNDM and all the patients carrying mutations in this gene were born from consanguineous marriage [34].

3.8.3 United Arab Emirates

The incidence estimated in the period 1985–2013 is at least 1 in 29,241 live births, with a rate of 1 in 31,900 for PNDM and 1 in 350,903 for TNDM. The genetic defect was identified in 84% of the probands. Interestingly, the 25 patients were born from 15 families and the most common cause was homozygous *EIF2AK3* mutations detected in nine patients (36%) from 5 families, followed by the recessive *INS* mutation (of note, the c-331C > G mutation in all of them) in 7 patients (28%). Consanguinity was detected in 88% of the study cohort [35].

3.8.4 Saudi Arabia

The only report from this Country was published in 2011 [36] and overviewed the patients with permanent neonatal diabetes born at or referred to the Al-Madinah Maternity and Children Hospital in the period from 2001 to 2010. Seventeen patients from 11 families were recruited with an incidence of 1 in 21,196 live births. Gene defects were identified in 14 of 17 patients (82.4%). Half of the 14 patients had Wolcott-Rallison syndrome and 5 of them (35.7%) had a mutation in the GLIS3 gene, showing also congenital hypothyroidism. Interestingly, also the remaining 2 patients presented syndromic diabetes (TRMA and Fanconi-Bickel syndrome). The incidence estimated in this Country is the highest ever reported and is due to the high consanguinity rate in that area (67.2%) and all the patients described were born from consanguineous marriages.

3.8.5 *Iran*

We have no data about incidence of NDM, but a 2019 report shows that Wolcott-Rallison syndrome accounts for about 22% of cases. In this Country, familial marriage is quite common (37.4%) and explains the frequency of such disease. The rate of consanguineous parents among these patients was 78.6%. In the same cohort, mutations in the KCNJ11, ABCC8, and INS genes altogether accounted for 31% of cases of NDM [37].

3.8.6 *Turkey*

The incidence of neonatal diabetes in the 4-year period (2010–2013) was 1 in 30,000 live births (PNDM 1 in 48,000) in the South-Eastern Anatolian region. Twenty-two patients were diagnosed in that period, 5 with transient and 17 with permanent NDM. A gene mutation was found in 20 patients (95% of the cohort), with 6q24 abnormalities as the most frequent genetic cause of TNDM (60%) and homozygous *GCK* mutations as the most frequent one for PNDM (35%) followed by homozygous mutations in *EIF2AK3* (17.5%) and in *PTF1A* (17.5%). The high detection rate (90%) as compared to other cohorts is likely due to genetic techniques, while the high rate of consanguinity in Turkey accounts for the high rate of homozygous mutations [38].

3.8.7 *Qatar*

The incidence in indigenous Qatari population is the second highest reported incidence after what was reported in Northwest Saudi Arabia. It has been estimated on a 16-year period of observation, from 2001 to 2016. Nine patients born from 7 first-degree consanguineous families were diagnosed with PNDM with an incidence of 1 in 22,938 live births among the indigenous Qatari population (43.6% for million of indigenous Qataris and 22.2 for million in non indigenous Qataris). These patients account for 12% of the diabetic population with diabetes onset within the first 5 years of life. No mutations in ABCC8 and KCNJ11 genes were found, while the most frequent cause of NDM was mutations in *PTF1A*, followed by INS gene mutations [39].

3.9 North America

3.9.1 *United States*

In 2008, a single center report from the University of Chicago described 32 consecutive patients with diabetes onset before 6 months and 45 with diabetes onset between 6 and 12 months of age. Interestingly, 85% of the patients were of

European descent. KCNJ11 gene mutations were found in 16 patients with onset in the first 6 months of life (50%) and none between 6 and 12 months of age, while INS gene mutations were detected in 4 patients with onset in the first 6 months of life (12.5%) and in 3 (6.7%) with onset at 6–12 months of age. No mutations in *ABCC8* were found. No other genes were screened [40]. Data about incidence in the period 2001–2008 are available from the SEARCH for Diabetes in Youth database, which is a multi-center study involving patients 0–19 years old with diabetes onset from Ohio, Washington, South Carolina, Colorado, Hawaii, and California. Forty patients out of 15,829 patients presented diabetes within the first 6 months of age (one of them was excluded from epidemiological evaluation because of secondary diabetes), hence the rate of NDM was 0.25%. PNDM was diagnosed in 35 patients (prevalence in SEARCH 0.22%), TNDM in 3 (prevalence in SEARCH 0.02%) (data not available for one patient). Unfortunately, only 8 patients were available for genetic testing and thus these data do not provide useful information about the prevalence of the different mutated genes. However, on the basis of these data, the prevalence of PNDM in youth was estimated to be 1 in 252,000 (1 in 145,000 in the prevalence 2001 cohort; 1 in 476,000 in the 2002–2008 incidence cohorts) [41].

3.10 Conclusions

These findings suggest that NDM has a different genetic aetiology compared to Japan, Europe, and the USA, clearly affected by consanguinity. Surprisingly, on the basis of the report from other Countries, 1–2 patients carrying a mutation in the "classical" neonatal diabetes genes, *KCNJ11*, *ABCC8*, and *INS* were expected, on the basis of live births, but not found. Data from a large national database show that it may occur in 3.3–47.2 live births for 1,000,000. It is more frequent in those Societies in whom consanguineous marriage is common. In these Countries homozygous or compound heterozygous mutations and rare syndromes associated with neonatal diabetes account for most of the patients. On the other hand, isolated neonatal diabetes and heterozygous mutations account are more commonly found.

3.11 Conclusion

Neonatal diabetes mellitus is a rare disease whose incidence has increased over the last three decades. There is no evidence to suggest that the true incidence of this disorder has become more frequent, but we are prone to suggest that different factors (laboratories facilities, increased awareness of its mechanisms, increased survival rate, and increased referral rate) have contributed to increase the number of diagnoses patients and thus to increase the estimated minimal incidence.

References

1. Pihoker C, Gilliam LK, Ellard S, Dabelea D, Davis C, Dolan LM, Greenbaum CJ, Imperatore G, Lawrence JM, Marcovina SM, Mayer-Davis E, Rodriguez BL, Steck AK, Williams DE, Hattersley AT, SEARCH for Diabetes in Youth Study Group. Prevalence, characteristics and clinical diagnosis of maturity onset diabetes of the young due to mutations in HNF1A, HNF4A, and glucokinase: results from the SEARCH for Diabetes in Youth. J Clin Endocrinol Metab. 2013;98(10):4055–62. https://doi.org/10.1210/jc.2013-1279.
2. Habeb AM, Flanagan SE, Deeb A, Al-Alwan I, Alawneh H, Balafrej AA, Mutair A, Hattersley AT, Hussain K, Ellard S. Permanent neonatal diabetes: different aetiology in Arabs compared to Europeans. Arch Dis Child. 2012;97(8):721–3. https://doi.org/10.1136/archdischild-2012-301744.
3. Gomella T, Eyal F, Bany-Mohammed F. Gomella's neonatology, 8th ed. 2020. McGraw-Hill. ISBN 9781259644818.
4. Von Muhlendahl KE, Herkenhoff H. Long-term course of neonatal diabetes. N Engl J Med. 1995;333:704–8.
5. Iafusco D, Stazi MA, Cotichini R, Cotellessa M, Martinucci ME, Mazzella M, Cherubini V, Barbetti F, Martinetti M, Cerutti F, Prisco F, the Early Onset Diabetes Study Group of the Italian Society of Paediatric Endocrinology and Diabetology. Permanent diabetes mellitus in the first year of life. Diabetologia. 2002;45:798–804.
6. Johnson MB, Hattersley AT, Flanagan SE. Monogenic autoimmune diseases of the endocrine system. Lancet Diabet Endocrinol. 2016;4:862–72.
7. Barbetti F, Mammì C, Liu M, Grasso V, Arvan P, Remedi M, Nichols C. Neonatal diabetes: permanent neonatal diabetes and transient neonatal diabetes. In: Diabetes associated with single gene defects and chromosomal abnormalities. F. Barbetti, L. Ghizzoni, F. Guaraldi, editors. Frontiers in diabetes, 2017;25:1-25; S. Karger AG: Basel. ISBN: 978-3-318-06024-9; ISSN: 02515342; https://doi.org/10.1159/isbn.978-3-318-06025-6
8. De Franco E. From biology to genes and back again: gene discovery for monogenic forms of beta-cell dysfunction and diabetes. J Mol Biol. 2020;432:1535–50.
9. Nansseu JR, Ngo-Um SS, Balti EV. Incidence, prevalence and genetic determinants of neonatal diabetes mellitus: a systematic review and meta-analysis protocol. Syst Rev. 2016;5(1):188. https://doi.org/10.1186/s13643-016-0369-3.
10. Saraswathi S, Al-Khawaga S, Elkum N, Hussain K. A systematic review of childhood diabetes research in the Middle East Region. Front Endocrinol (Lausanne). 2019;10:805. https://doi.org/10.3389/fendo.2019.00805.
11. Imerslund O. The prognosis in diabetes with onset before age two. Acta Paediatr. 1960;49:243–8. https://doi.org/10.1111/j.1651-2227.1960.tb07730.x.
12. Fösel S. Transient and permanent neonatal diabetes. Eur J Pediatr. 1995;154(12):944–8. https://doi.org/10.1007/BF01958635.
13. Jefferson IG, Smith MA, Baum JD. Insulin dependent diabetes in under 5 year olds. Arch Dis Child. 1985;60(12):1144–8. https://doi.org/10.1136/adc.60.12.1144.
14. Rosenbauer J, Herzig P, von Kries R, Neu A, Giani G. Temporal, seasonal, and geographical incidence patterns of Type I diabetes mellitus in children under 5 years of age in Germany. Diabetologia. 1999;42:1055–9.
15. Iafusco D, Stazi MA, Cotichini R, Cotellessa M, Martinucci ME, Mazzella M, Cherubini V, Barbetti F, Martinetti M, Cerutti F, Prisco F, Early Onset Diabetes Study Group of the Italian Society of Paediatric Endocrinology and Diabetology. Permanent diabetes mellitus in the first year of life. Diabetologia. 2002;45(6):798–804. https://doi.org/10.1007/s00125-002-0837-2.
16. Pacaud D, Schwandt A, de Beaufort C, Casteels K, Beltrand J, Birkebaek NH, Campagnoli M, Bratina N, Limbert C, Mp O'Riordan S, Ribeiro R, Gerasimidi-Vazeou A, Petruzelkova L, Verkauskiene R, Krisane ID, SWEET Study Group. A description of clinician reported diagnosis of type 2 diabetes and other non-type 1 diabetes included in a large international mul-

ticentered pediatric diabetes registry (SWEET). Pediatr Diabetes. 2016;17(Suppl 23):24–31. https://doi.org/10.1111/pedi.12426.
17. Slingerland AS, Shields BM, Flanagan SE, Bruining GJ, Noordam K, Gach A, Mlynarski W, Malecki MT, Hattersley AT, Ellard S. Referral rates for diagnostic testing support an incidence of permanent neonatal diabetes in three European countries of at least 1 in 260,000 live births. Diabetologia. 2009;52(8):1683–5. https://doi.org/10.1007/s00125-009-1416-6.
18. Busiah K, Drunat S, Vaivre-Douret L, Bonnefond A, Simon A, Flechtner I, Gérard B, Pouvreau N, Elie C, Nimri R, De Vries L, Tubiana-Rufi N, Metz C, Bertrand AM, Nivot-Adamiak S, de Kerdanet M, Stuckens C, Jennane F, Souchon PF, Le Tallec C, Désirée C, Pereira S, Dechaume A, Robert JJ, Phillip M, Scharfmann R, Czernichow P, Froguel P, Vaxillaire M, Polak M, Cavé H, French NDM study group. Neuropsychological dysfunction and developmental defects associated with genetic changes in infants with neonatal diabetes mellitus: a prospective cohort study [corrected]. Lancet Diabetes Endocrinol. 2013;1(3):199–207. https://doi.org/10.1016/S2213-8587(13)70059-7.
19. Fendler W, Borowiec M, Baranowska-Jazwiecka A, Szadkowska A, Skala-Zamorowska E, Deja G, Jarosz-Chobot P, Techmanska I, Bautembach-Minkowska J, Mysliwiec M, Zmyslowska A, Pietrzak I, Malecki MT, Mlynarski W. Prevalence of monogenic diabetes amongst Polish children after a nationwide genetic screening campaign. Diabetologia. 2012;55(10):2631–5. https://doi.org/10.1007/s00125-012-2621-2.
20. Małachowska B, Borowiec M, Antosik K, Michalak A, Baranowska-Jaźwiecka A, Deja G, Jarosz-Chobot P, Brandt A, Myśliwiec M, Stelmach M, Nazim J, Peczyńska J, Głowińska-Olszewska B, Horodnicka-Józwa A, Walczak M, Małecki MT, Zmysłowska A, Szadkowska A, Fendler W, Młynarski W. Monogenic diabetes prevalence among polish children-summary of 11 years-long nationwide genetic screening program. Pediatr Diabetes. 2018;19(1):53–8. https://doi.org/10.1111/pedi.12532.
21. Grulich-Henn J, Wagner V, Thon A, Schober E, Marg W, Kapellen TM, Haberland H, Raile K, Ellard S, Flanagan SE, Hattersley AT, Holl RW. Entities and frequency of neonatal diabetes: data from the diabetes documentation and quality management system (DPV). Diabet Med. 2010;27(6):709–12. https://doi.org/10.1111/j.1464-5491.2010.02965.x.
22. Wiedemann B, Schober E, Waldhoer T, Koehle J, Flanagan SE, Mackay DJ, Steichen E, Meraner D, Zimmerhackl LB, Hattersley AT, Ellard S, Hofer S. Incidence of neonatal diabetes in Austria-calculation based on the Austrian Diabetes Register. Pediatr Diabetes. 2010;11(1):18–23. https://doi.org/10.1111/j.1399-5448.2009.00530.x.
23. Iafusco D, Massa O, Pasquino B, Colombo C, Iughetti L, Bizzarri C, Mammì C, Lo Presti D, Suprani T, Schiaffini R, Nichols CG, Russo L, Grasso V, Meschi F, Bonfanti R, Brescianini S, Barbetti F, Early Diabetes Study Group of ISPED. Minimal incidence of neonatal/infancy onset diabetes in Italy is 1:90,000 live births. Acta Diabetol. 2012;49(5):405–8. https://doi.org/10.1007/s00592-011-0331-8.
24. Russo L, Iafusco D, Brescianini S, Nocerino V, Bizzarri C, Toni S, Cerutti F, Monciotti C, Pesavento R, Iughetti L, Bernardini L, Bonfanti R, Gargantini L, Vanelli M, Aguilar-Bryan L, Stazi MA, Grasso V, Colombo C, Barbetti F, ISPED Early Diabetes Study Group. Permanent diabetes during the first year of life: multiple gene screening in 54 patients. Diabetologia. 2011;54(7):1693–701. https://doi.org/10.1007/s00125-011-2094-8.
25. Delvecchio M, Mozzillo E, Salzano G, Iafusco D, Frontino G, Patera PI, Rabbone I, Cherubini V, Grasso V, Tinto N, Giglio S, Contreas G, Di Paola R, Salina A, Cauvin V, Tumini S, d'Annunzio G, Iughetti L, Mantovani V, Maltoni G, Toni S, Marigliano M, Barbetti F; Diabetes Study Group of the Italian Society of Pediatric Endocrinology and Diabetes (ISPED). Monogenic diabetes accounts for 6.3% of cases referred to 15 Italian pediatric diabetes centers during 2007 to 2012. J Clin Endocrinol Metab. 2017;102(6):1826–1834. https://doi.org/10.1210/jc.2016-2490.
26. Stanik J, Gasperikova D, Paskova M, Barak L, Javorkova J, Jancova E, Ciljakova M, Hlava P, Michalek J, Flanagan SE, Pearson E, Hattersley AT, Ellard S, Klimes I. Prevalence of permanent neonatal diabetes in Slovakia and successful replacement of insulin with sulfonylurea therapy

in KCNJ11 and ABCC8 mutation carriers. J Clin Endocrinol Metab. 2007;92(4):1276–82. https://doi.org/10.1210/jc.2006-2490.
27. Globa E, Zelinska N, Mackay DJ, Temple KI, Houghton JA, Hattersley AT, Flanagan SE, Ellard S. Neonatal diabetes in Ukraine: incidence, genetics, clinical phenotype and treatment. J Pediatr Endocrinol Metab. 2015;28(11–12):1279–86. https://doi.org/10.1515/jpem-2015-0170.
28. Cao B, Gong C, Wu D, Lu C, Liu F, Liu X, Zhang Y, Gu Y, Qi Z, Li X, Liu M, Li W, Su C, Liang X, Feng M. Genetic analysis and follow-up of 25 neonatal diabetes mellitus patients in China. J Diabetes Res. 2016;2016:6314368. https://doi.org/10.1155/2016/6314368.
29. Nagashima K, Tanaka D, Inagaki N. Epidemiology, clinical characteristics, and genetic etiology of neonatal diabetes in Japan. Pediatr Int. 2017;59(2):129–33. https://doi.org/10.1111/ped.13199.
30. Suzuki S, Makita Y, Mukai T, Matsuo K, Ueda O, Fujieda K. Molecular basis of neonatal diabetes in Japanese patients. J Clin Endocrinol Metab. 2007;92(10):3979–85. https://doi.org/10.1210/jc.2007-0486.
31. Ogle GD, Morrison MK, Silink M, Taito RS. Incidence and prevalence of diabetes in children aged <15 yr in Fiji, 2001-2012. Pediatr Diabetes. 2016;17(3):222–6. https://doi.org/10.1111/pedi.12257.
32. Soliman AT, el Zalabany MM, Bappal B, al Salmi I, de Silva V, Asfour M. Permanent neonatal diabetes mellitus: epidemiology, mode of presentation, pathogenesis and growth. Indian J Pediatr. 1999;66(3):363–73. https://doi.org/10.1007/BF02845526.
33. Al Senani A, Hamza N, Al Azkawi H, Al Kharusi M, Al Sukaiti N, Al Badi M, Al Yahyai M, Johnson M, De Franco E, Flanagan S, Hattersley A, Ellard S, Mula-Abed WA. Genetic mutations associated with neonatal diabetes mellitus in Omani patients. J Pediatr Endocrinol Metab. 2018;31(2):195–204. https://doi.org/10.1515/jpem-2017-0284.
34. Abujbara MA, Liswi MI, El-Khateeb MS, Flanagan SE, Ellard S, Ajlouni KM. Permanent neonatal diabetes mellitus in Jordan. J Pediatr Endocrinol Metab. 2014;27(9–10):879–83. https://doi.org/10.1515/jpem-2014-0069.
35. Deeb A, Kaplan W, Attia S, Hadi S, Osman A, Al-Jubeh J, Flanagan S, De Franco E, Ellard S. Genetic characteristics, clinical spectrum, and incidence of neonatal diabetes in the Emirate of Abu Dhabi, United Arab Emirates. Am J Med Genet A. 2016;170(3):602–9. https://doi.org/10.1002/ajmg.a.37419.
36. Habeb AM, Al-Magamsi MS, Eid IM, Ali MI, Hattersley AT, Hussain K, Ellard S. Incidence, genetics, and clinical phenotype of permanent neonatal diabetes mellitus in Northwest Saudi Arabia. Pediatr Diabetes. 2012;13(6):499–505. https://doi.org/10.1111/j.1399-5448.2011.00828.x.
37. Asl SN, Vakili R, Vakili S, Soheilipour F, Hashemipour M, Ghahramani S, De Franco E, Yaghootkar H. Wolcott-Rallison syndrome in Iran: a common cause of neonatal diabetes. J Pediatr Endocrinol Metab. 2019;32(6):607–13. https://doi.org/10.1515/jpem-2018-0434.
38. Demirbilek H, Arya VB, Ozbek MN, Houghton JA, Baran RT, Akar M, Tekes S, Tuzun H, Mackay DJ, Flanagan SE, Hattersley AT, Ellard S, Hussain K. Clinical characteristics and molecular genetic analysis of 22 patients with neonatal diabetes from the South-Eastern region of Turkey: predominance of non-KATP channel mutations. Eur J Endocrinol. 2015;172(6):697–705. https://doi.org/10.1530/EJE-14-0852.
39. Al-Khawaga S, Mohammed I, Saraswathi S, Haris B, Hasnah R, Saeed A, Almabrazi H, Syed N, Jithesh P, El Awwa A, Khalifa A, AlKhalaf F, Petrovski G, Abdelalim EM, Hussain K. The clinical and genetic characteristics of permanent neonatal diabetes (PNDM) in the state of Qatar. Mol Genet Genomic Med. 2019;7(10):e00753. https://doi.org/10.1002/mgg3.753.
40. Støy J, Greeley SA, Paz VP, Ye H, Pastore AN, Skowron KB, Lipton RB, Cogen FR, Bell GI. Philipson LH; United States neonatal diabetes working group. Diagnosis and treatment of neonatal diabetes: a United States experience. Pediatr Diabetes. 2008 Oct;9(5):450–9. https://doi.org/10.1111/j.1399-5448.2008.00433.x.

41. Kanakatti Shankar R, Pihoker C, Dolan LM, Standiford D, Badaru A, Dabelea D, Rodriguez B, Black MH, Imperatore G, Hattersley A, Ellard S, Gilliam LK, SEARCH for Diabetes in Youth Study Group. Permanent neonatal diabetes mellitus: prevalence and genetic diagnosis in the SEARCH for Diabetes in Youth Study. Pediatr Diabetes. 2013;14(3):174–80. https://doi.org/10.1111/pedi.12003.

Chapter 4
Classification of Neonatal Diabetes

Elisa De Franco and Matthew B. Johnson

4.1 Neonatal Diabetes

Neonatal Diabetes Mellitus (NDM) is defined as hyperglycemia presenting in the first 6 months of life, persisting for over 2 weeks and requiring treatment. Two separate studies [1, 2] have shown that diabetes diagnosed before 6 months of age is most likely to have a monogenic cause rather than being polygenic type 1 diabetes.

In this chapter, we discuss the classification of neonatal and early-onset subtypes according to clinical and genetic features.

4.2 Clinical Classification

Based on the diabetes progression and the presence or absence of other features, NDM has been traditionally classified into three groups: PNDM, TNDM, and syndromic NDM.

Supplementary Information The online version contains supplementary material available at https://doi.org/10.1007/978-3-031-07008-2_4.

E. De Franco (✉) · M. B. Johnson
Institute of Biomedical and Clinical Sciences, University of Exeter College of Medicine and Health, Exeter, UK
e-mail: E.De-Franco@exeter.ac.uk; M.Johnson@exeter.ac.uk

I. Rabbone, D. Iafusco (eds.), *Neonatal and Early Onset Diabetes Mellitus*,
https://doi.org/10.1007/978-3-031-07008-2_4

4.2.1 Transient Neonatal Diabetes

Transient Neonatal Diabetes (TNDM) is characterized by onset in the first 6 months of life with persistent hyperglycemia requiring treatment. The insulin requirement progressively reduces in these patients and diabetes remits usually before the age of 5 years [3]. Individuals with TNDM typically live diabetes-free for months to years, but in 40% the diabetes relapses later in life [4].

4.2.2 Permanent Neonatal Diabetes

PNDM is estimated to account for approximately half of NDM cases. It presents in the first 6 months of life and requires treatment throughout the patients' lifespan. While originally all patients with PNDM would have been treated with insulin, the identification of activating mutations in the beta-cell potassium channel genes *ABCC8* and *KCNJ11* in the early 2000s (see below) as major causes of PNDM resulted in many of these patients being able to transfer from insulin injections to sulfonylurea tablets, with improved glucose control and quality of life [5–8].

4.2.3 Syndromic Neonatal and Early-Onset Diabetes

PNDM can present as part of a multi-system syndrome. Since PNDM is diagnosed in the first 6 months of life, it is often the presenting feature in syndromic NDM subtypes [9]. Before the availability of early comprehensive genetic testing, patients would traditionally be classified as having PNDM until presentation of other features would prompt reclassification to one of the recognized syndromes including NDM.

A subset of patients with PNDM are born with absent (or very small) pancreas, a condition called pancreatic agenesis (also referred to as pancreatic hypoplasia). These patients are typically born small for gestational age and are diagnosed with diabetes in the first weeks of life. As a result of pancreatic development failure, these individuals also have exocrine pancreatic insufficiency requiring oral supplementation therapy [10]. Recognition and treatment of these patients' exocrine deficiency are essential to avoid severe growth delay. Pancreatic agenesis/hypoplasia can be identified through imaging (ultrasound or MRI scan), however, this is often challenging in small babies. Measurement of fecal elastase (low or undetectable in these patients) is a more practical approach in neonates with NDM to detect exocrine pancreatic insufficiency and clinically diagnose pancreatic agenesis.

4.3 Genetic and Biological Classification

As of 2021, 32 genetic subtypes of NDM have been reported in at least 2 unrelated families. The genetic heterogeneity of NDM highlights different biological mechanisms which, when disrupted, can result in beta-cell dysfunction soon after birth and development of NDM (Fig. 4.1). In this chapter, we grouped the known genetic causes of NDM into 7 categories based on their likely effect on beta-cells and we discuss genetic and clinical features of each subtype in the sections below.

4.3.1 Defects in Glucose Sensing/Insulin Secretion

The primary function of the insulin-producing beta-cells is to produce and release insulin in response to glucose. It is, therefore, not surprising that any disruption to the pathway linking glucose sensing to insulin production and release would result in the inability of beta-cells to release insulin and diabetes onset in the neonatal period. So far, pathogenic mutations in 6 genes involved in this essential biological pathway have been found to cause NDM/early-onset diabetes.

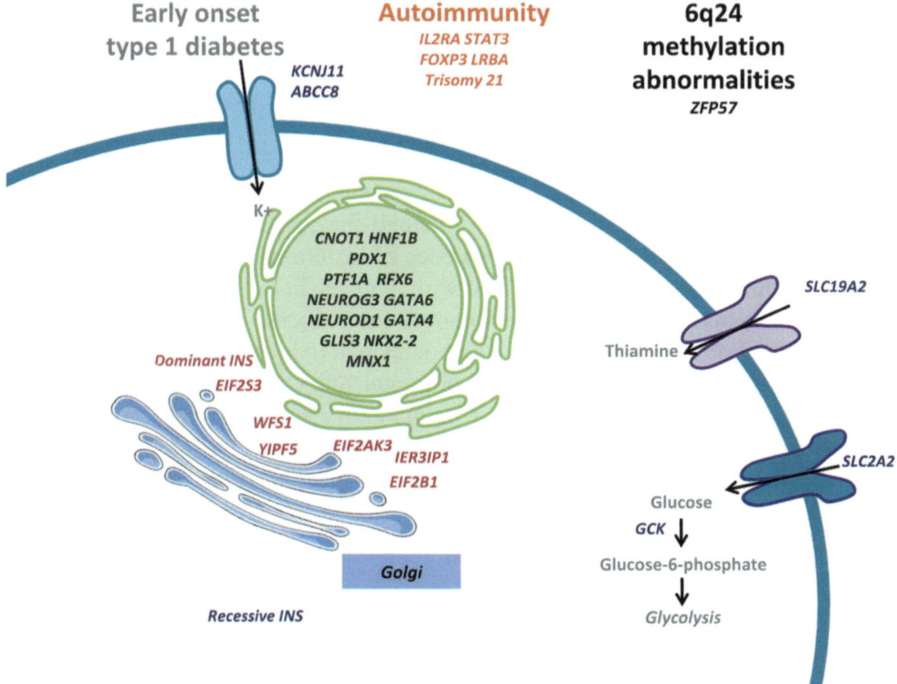

Fig. 4.1 Schematic representation of the 32 genetic causes resulting in NDM through seven different mechanisms

4.3.1.1 Neonatal Diabetes Caused by Activating *KCNJ11* and *ABCC8* Mutations

The most common causes of NDM, identified in approximately 40% of patients [9], are activating mutations in the *KCNJ11* and *ABCC8* genes encoding the two beta-cell potassium channel subunits [5, 11, 12]. These mutations can cause transient neonatal/adult-onset diabetes, PNDM, or DEND (Developmental delay Epilepsy and Neonatal Diabetes) syndrome [3, 5, 6, 11, 12]. Electrophysiology studies have shown that the phenotype severity is directly correlated to the severity of the mutation [13]. More recent studies have suggested that all patients with activating *ABCC8* and *KCNJ11* mutations—even those not diagnosed with DEND or intermediate DEND syndrome—may have some degree of neurological involvement, with developmental coordination disorder or attention deficits being often detected following in-depth neuro-psychomotor assessments [14, 15]. An early genetic diagnosis is essential in patients with NDM caused by activating *ABCC8* or *KCNJ11* mutations as most of them achieve improved glycemic control after transfer from insulin to sulfonylurea therapy [7, 8] which has been shown to be effective long-term [16, 17]. Treatment with sulfonylurea also improves neurological outcomes and some studies have suggested that early treatment may be most beneficial for the patients' neurodevelopment. While mutations in *KCNJ11* are always dominantly acting, mutations in *ABCC8* can act as either dominant or recessive and are often inherited [13].

4.3.1.2 Neonatal Diabetes Caused by Autosomal Recessive *INS* Mutations

Inactivation of both alleles of the insulin (*INS*) gene causes NDM. Patients with this genetic subtype of NDM are usually born small for gestational age (median birth weight Z score—3.2) [18], reflecting absence of insulin-mediated growth in utero. These individuals are usually diagnosed with diabetes in the first month of life and require insulin treatment [18]. While homozygous nonsense and splicing mutations result in PNDM, homozygous and compound heterozygous mutations affecting critical nucleotides within the *INS* gene promoter often result in TNDM, with diabetes remission occurring in infancy [18]. Diabetes relapse has been reported, but the rate of diabetes relapse in this cohort is not known at present. Additional clinical features are very rare in patients with this subtype of NDM and are usually coincidental.

4.3.1.3 Neonatal Diabetes Caused by Autosomal Recessive *GCK* Mutations

Biallelic mutations resulting in loss of function of the *GCK* gene, encoding for the enzyme glucokinase, are a cause of PNDM [19]. Glucokinase is the beta-cell glucose sensor and heterozygous mutations are known to cause fasting hyperglycemia from birth (GCK-MODY), which does not require any treatment. In contrast, biallelic mutations result in insulin-dependent NDM [20]. These patients are usually born small for gestational age and develop diabetes in the neonatal period. Some patients who develop diabetes outside the neonatal period, predominantly in infancy, have also been reported with strong evidence of a genotype–phenotype correlation [21]. Similarly to individuals with biallelic *INS* mutations, these patients usually have no additional syndromic features [19]. Although the genetic diagnosis of PNDM, subtype GCK does not result in treatment change for the patient, it is important to highlight the possibility of GCK-MODY in family members, which are often mistakenly diagnosed as having type 1 diabetes and on the wrong treatment.

4.3.1.4 Neonatal Diabetes Caused by Autosomal Recessive *SLC2A2* Mutations (Fanconi-Bickel Syndrome)

Biallelic loss of function mutations in the glucose transporter gene *SLC2A2* [22] cause Fanconi-Bickel syndrome, a condition characterized by hepatorenal glycogen accumulation, renal dysfunction, and impaired utilization of glucose and galactose. Various additional features have been described, including TNDM [23]. *SLC2A2* mutations are a rare cause of neonatal diabetes, estimated to account for 0.6% of cases [9].

4.3.1.5 Neonatal Diabetes Caused by Autosomal Recessive *SLC19A2* Mutations (Thiamine Responsive Megaloblastic Anemia—TRMA—Syndrome, also Called Roger's Syndrome)

Biallelic loss of function mutations in *SLC19A2* cause TRMA syndrome [24]. These patients usually develop diabetes in childhood, but some individuals are diagnosed with diabetes in the neonatal period [25–27]. Treatment with thiamine results in resolution of anemia and transfusion independence and can also lead to improved glycemic control, with some patients becoming insulin independent [28]. While *SLC19A2* mutations are a relatively rare cause of neonatal diabetes (~0.7% of cases [9]), it is important to consider this diagnosis and test the gene in patients with NDM (especially when anemia and/or deafness are also present) as it could result in improved treatment and better disease outcome.

4.3.2 Beta-Cell Development

Mutations in genes involved in beta-cell development and maturation can result in NDM through a severely reduced number of mature beta-cells. These genes are all developmental transcription regulators, either involved in regulation of the developing pancreas (in which case mutations may result in pancreatic agenesis/hypoplasia) or in the formation and maturation of beta-cells specifically, in which case the mutations results in NDM without affecting pancreatic exocrine function.

4.3.2.1 Neonatal Diabetes Caused by Failure of Pancreatic Development

Mutations in seven transcription regulators which are essential at different stages of pancreatic development have been reported to cause pancreatic agenesis/hypoplasia, characterized by NDM and exocrine pancreatic insufficiency [29]. An early genetic diagnosis is essential to prompt investigation of their exocrine pancreatic function, as oral replacement therapy is often needed and is important to prevent growth delay.

Neonatal Diabetes Caused by Autosomal Recessive *PDX1* Mutations

Autosomal recessive mutations in the *PDX1* (also known as *IPF1*) gene were the first reported cause of isolated pancreatic agenesis [30, 31]. However, the phenotypic spectrum of diabetes associated with biallelic *PDX1* missense mutations is broad with some patients having PNDM and subclinical exocrine insufficiency [32] or isolated PNDM with normal exocrine function [33].

Neonatal Diabetes Caused by Autosomal Recessive *PTF1A* Mutations

Homozygous protein-truncating mutations in *PTF1A* cause PNDM due to pancreatic agenesis, severe intrauterine growth retardation (IUGR), microcephaly, and cerebellar hypoplasia/agenesis [34]. The condition is usually lethal within the first few weeks of life. In 2014, Weedon et al. reported biallelic mutations in a distal *PTF1A* enhancer in 10 families with pancreatic agenesis but no additional neurological features [35]. Functional studies showed that the enhancer was pancreatic-specific and active during differentiation of pancreatic progenitors. A recent report of 30 patients with biallelic *PTF1A* enhancer mutations observed that, while none of the patients had the severe neurological features reported in patients with coding loss of function mutations, additional features such as growth retardation, anemia, and cholestasis were common [36]. Homozygosity for the *PTF1A* missense mutation, p.(Pro191Thr), also causes pancreatic agenesis without additional neurological features [37]. In vitro studies showed that this mutation likely results in partial loss of function, thus explaining the "milder" phenotype observed in patients with this variant compared to the other reported coding mutations [37].

Neonatal Diabetes Caused by Autosomal Dominant *HNF1B* Mutations

Heterozygous loss of function mutations and deletions resulting in haploinsufficiency of the *HNF1B* gene cause a multi-developmental disorder known as Renal Cysts and Diabetes Syndrome (RCAD) . Patients with RCAD syndrome usually develop diabetes outside the neonatal period, after presentation of renal disease [38]. Pancreatic atrophy and defects of pancreatic exocrine function are common in patients with *HNF1B* mutations and deletions, suggesting a defect in pancreatic development [39]. Heterozygous *HNF1B* mutations can sometimes cause NDM, with two cases reported in the literature [40, 41]. In both previously reported cases, after an initial diagnosis in the first month of life, insulin requirement decreased, with insulin treatment becoming intermittent in one case and interrupted in the second patient. In both cases, diabetes relapsed in infancy. The patient reported by Edghill et al. [41] had marked pancreatic atrophy and further investigations confirmed subclinical exocrine as well as endocrine dysfunction. *HNF1B* mutations are therefore a rare cause of TNDM, and they are more often associated with early-onset diabetes and various degrees of renal dysfunction.

Neonatal Diabetes Caused by Autosomal Recessive *RFX6* Mutations (Mitchell-Riley Syndrome)

Biallelic loss of function mutations in the *RFX6* gene cause a syndrome featuring neonatal/early-onset diabetes, small bowel obstruction because of bowel atresia, and gallbladder agenesis/hypoplasia [42, 43]. These patients usually present with IUGR, hyperglycemia in the first days of life requiring insulin treatment, and intestinal atresia. Some patients also have an annular pancreas and exocrine pancreatic insufficiency. While the condition is sometimes lethal before the first year of life, follow-up studies suggested that patients who survive the first critical months of life have a good prognosis, with good management of their diabetes and normal development [44]. Heterozygous *RFX6* mutations cause adult-onset diabetes, therefore parents of children with *RFX6*-NDM should be monitored [45].

Neonatal Diabetes Caused by Autosomal Dominant Mutations in *GATA6*

Heterozygous loss of function mutations in *GATA6* cause a wide spectrum of developmental defects. *GATA6* mutations were first reported to cause congenital heart defects [46]. Subsequently, investigations into novel genetic causes of syndromic pancreatic genesis identified mutations in *GATA6* as the most common cause of pancreatic agenesis in humans [10]. Patients with *GATA6*-NDM usually have additional extra-pancreatic features, including congenital heart defects, hepatobiliary malformations, particularly gallbladder agenesis, and gut abnormalities. A later study showed that mutations in *GATA6* are associated with a wide spectrum of diabetes phenotypes, including TNDM and adult-onset diabetes without exocrine pancreatic insufficiency [47].

Neonatal and Early-Onset Diabetes Caused by Autosomal Dominant Mutations in *GATA4*

Haploinsufficiency of *GATA4* is a known cause of congenital heart defects [48, 49]. Two studies have reported three cases with heterozygous mutations in *GATA4* and pancreatic agenesis: two of these patients also had congenital heart defects [48–51]. One of the studies reported two additional patients with deletions including *GATA4* who had diabetes diagnosed in early infancy but normal exocrine function [51]. This suggests that mutations in *GATA4* are associated with a more variable phenotype than *GATA6* and are a much rarer cause of pancreatic agenesis.

Neonatal Diabetes Caused by a Specific Heterozygous *CNOT1* Mutation

Four patients with the same heterozygous *CNOT1* missense mutation, p.(Arg535Cys), and pancreatic agenesis have been reported by two studies [29, 52]. The mutation had arisen de novo in all cases where both parental samples were available for testing. Three of these patients also had holoprosencephaly and the fourth had facial features potentially consistent with holoprosencephaly but a brain scan was not available. A fifth patient with holoprosencephaly but without NDM was also reported [52]. While a very rare cause of pancreatic agenesis, the identification of this *CNOT1* mutation was important to further highlight the mechanisms regulating pancreatic development, as CNOT1 had never before been suspected to be important for pancreatic development.

4.3.2.2 Neonatal Diabetes Caused by Failure of Beta-Cell Development

Mutations resulting in the disruption of at least five genes involved in the transcriptional pathway regulating beta-cell development, from the differentiation of endocrine progenitors to generation of mature insulin-producing beta-cells, have been reported to cause syndromic forms of NDM.

Neonatal Diabetes Caused by Autosomal Recessive *GLIS3* Mutations (NDH Syndrome)

Biallelic loss of function mutations in *GLIS3* cause NDH syndrome (neonatal diabetes and hypothyroidism) [53]. Over 15 patients have been reported so far, all with a very consistent phenotype of IUGR, diabetes diagnosed in the first month of life and congenital hypothyroidism [54–56]. Hepatic and renal diseases and characteristic facial features have also been reported to be common [55, 57]. The majority of patients reported so far harbor deletions involving one or more of the 11 *GLIS3* exons, however, protein truncating and missense mutations affecting the DNA-binding domain have also been reported [55].

Neonatal Diabetes Caused by Autosomal Recessive *NEUROD1* Mutations

Homozygous mutations in *NEUROD1* have been reported in three families [58, 59]. All three infants were diagnosed with PNDM in the first 10 weeks of life; they presented with IUGR and had multiple neurological features (including developmental delay, sensorineural deafness, myopia, and diffuse retinal dystrophy). Two cases were homozygous for frameshift mutations predicted to result in a truncated protein lacking the transactivation domain, while the third was a missense mutation affecting the DNA binding domain, suggesting that all three variants result in loss of NEUROD1 function.

Neonatal Diabetes Caused by Autosomal Recessive *NEUROG3* Mutations

Homozygous *NEUROG3* was initially found to cause Congenital malabsorptive diarrhea, with two out of three patients developing diabetes at the age of 8 years (the third patient died during childhood) [60]. Subsequently, 4 cases with biallelic *NEUROG3* missense and frameshift mutations who developed PNDM in addition to enteric anendocrinosis and malabsorptive diarrhea were reported [61–63]. Similar to other patients with NDM caused by mutations in genes regulating beta-cell development, these individuals were born small for gestational age and developed diabetes in the first month of life. The difference in age at onset of diabetes in patients with biallelic *NEUROG3* mutations was initially thought to be dependent on genotype, with complete loss of function mutations resulting in NDM and “hypomorphic” missense pathogenic variants causing infancy-onset diabetes. However, a recent report of two patients with biallelic loss of function *NEUROG3* mutations who developed diabetes at the ages 3 and 7 years, suggests that the phenotypic variability is not completely explained by the genotype [64].

Neonatal Diabetes Caused by Autosomal Recessive *NKX2–2* Mutations

Biallelic loss of function *NKX2-2* mutations are a rare cause of PNDM which has so far been reported in 4 patients from 3 unrelated families [65, 66]. These patients all presented with severe IUGR and PNDM with onset in the first week of life. All patients had moderate or severe developmental delay and hypoplastic corpus callosum was noted in one patient [66]. A recent report suggested that patients with this subtype of NDM develop severe infantile-onset obesity [65]. All patients reported so far harbored truncating mutations resulting in likely loss of function of the NKX2-2 protein.

Neonatal Diabetes Caused by Autosomal Recessive *MNX1* Mutations

Heterozygous loss of function mutations in *MNX1* are known to cause Currarino syndrome, a multisystem disorder that does not include NDM [67]. Two homozygous missense mutations affecting the MNX1 protein's DNA binding domain have been reported in two unrelated patients diagnosed with PNDM [66, 68]. Additional features similar to those identified in patients with Currarino syndrome, such as developmental delay, neurogenic bladder, and sacral agenesis were reported in one patient who died at the age of 10 months. The other patient, who was diagnosed with diabetes at the age of 1 day, was not reported to have additional extra-pancreatic features. Since only two patients have been reported so far, it is unclear whether *MNX1* mutations cause isolated PNDM, syndromic NDM, or both. Identification of other patients will be essential to define the clinical phenotype of this rare NDM subtype.

4.3.3 Non-autoimmune Beta-Cell Death

Mutations in genes affecting beta-cell survival are a common cause of both isolated and syndromic PNDM. All these mutations result in beta-cell death by altering the beta-cell response to endoplasmic reticulum (ER) stress. In contrast to NDM patients with gene mutations affecting pancreatic development, individuals with mutations resulting in beta-cell death through ER stress do not have severe IUGR at birth and are typically diagnosed later in the neonatal period (between 3 and 6 months), or sometimes outside the neonatal period.

4.3.3.1 Neonatal Diabetes Caused by Autosomal Dominant *INS* Mutations

Heterozygous mutations in the *INS* gene resulting in protein misfolding are a common cause of isolated PNDM [69], accounting for ~10% of cases born to non-consanguineous parents. These mutations usually occur in critical regions of the preproinsulin protein, likely resulting in accumulation of misfolded protein in the ER, triggering ER stress, and destruction of beta-cells through apoptosis. Although the vast majority of patients with heterozygous *INS* mutations have PNDM, diabetes onset in infancy and adulthood has also been reported [69].

4.3.3.2 Neonatal Diabetes Caused by Autosomal Recessive *EIF2AK3* Mutation (Wolcott-Rallison Syndrome)

The most common cause of PNDM among consanguineous patients is biallelic mutations in the *EIF2AK3* gene which cause Wolcott-Rallison Syndrome [70, 71]. *EIF2AK3* encodes PERK which is one of the ER sensors that regulate the unfolded protein response (UPR) [70]. The main features of Wolcott-Rallison Syndrome are neonatal/early-onset diabetes, skeletal dysplasia, and liver dysfunction [72], but additional features such as exocrine insufficiency, renal failure, hypothyroidism, and developmental delay can also be present. Wolcott-Rallison Syndrome usually has a poor prognosis, with most patients dying in infancy because of liver failure. Successful liver transplantation has been reported in one individual with Wolcott-Rallison syndrome. At the age of 8 years, 6 years after the transplant, this patient's diabetes was well controlled. However, skeletal dysplasia was found to progressively worsen over time [73]. Multi-organ transplant of liver, pancreas, and kidneys has been reported in three patients with Wolcott-Rallison syndrome, with good outcomes for some of the most life-threatening features of this condition [74–76].

4.3.3.3 Neonatal Diabetes Caused by Autosomal Recessive Mutations in *IER3IP1* (Microcephaly, Epilepsy, and Diabetes Syndrome 1; MEDS1)

Homozygous mutations affecting the *IER3IP1* gene have been found to cause MEDS (Microcephaly with simplified gyration, Epilepsy, and permanent neonatal Diabetes Syndrome) with 8 individuals reported so far [77–80]. Prognosis was generally poor, with 7/8 patients dying in infancy [80]. While the function of this gene is not entirely clear yet, it is likely that the *IER3IP1* mutations result in increased apoptosis, possibly through a similar pathway to Wolcott-Rallison syndrome [77].

4.3.3.4 Neonatal and Early-Onset Diabetes Caused by X-Linked Mutations in *EIF2S3* (MEHMO Syndrome)

Skopkova and colleagues reported *EIF2S3* pathogenic variants in three patients with X-linked MEHMO syndrome (a complex disease including mental retardation, epileptic seizures, hypogonadism and hypogenitalism, microcephaly, obesity) and neonatal/early-onset diabetes (two patients were diagnosed at 10 months and a third at 6 months) [81]. *EIF2S3* encodes for one of the subunits of the eukaryotic initiation factor 2 (eIF-2) and is therefore involved in the early steps of protein synthesis and ER stress regulation [81].

4.3.3.5 Neonatal and Early-Onset Diabetes Caused by Autosomal Dominant *WFS1* Mutations

Biallelic loss of function mutations in *WFS1* are a cause of Wolfram syndrome, a degenerative condition characterized by early-onset diabetes [82]. Diabetes is often the presenting feature, with other features such as optic atrophy, diabetes insipidus, and deafness developing in infancy through adulthood. More recently, heterozygous *de novo* mutations were reported to cause a congenital syndrome of neonatal/

early-onset diabetes, congenital cataracts, sensorineural deafness, hypotonia, and dysmorphic features [83]. The patients were diagnosed with diabetes between 3 and 12 months of age and all had additional features diagnosed at birth. Functional studies suggested that the *WFS1* mutations causing this syndromic form of NDM are likely to have a dominant-negative effect.

4.3.3.6 Neonatal and Early-Onset Diabetes Caused by Autosomal Dominant *EIF2B1* Mutations

Biallelic loss of function mutations in *EIF2B1* cause a rare neurological disorder, Leukoencephalopathy with vanishing white matter, which does not usually include diabetes [84]. However, heterozygous *EIF2B1* mutations which specifically result in loss of sensitivity of the EIF2B complex to eIF2α phosphorylation during the ER stress response, have been found to result in neonatal/early-onset diabetes (age at diagnosis range 4–56 weeks) in 5 unrelated patients [85]. The mutation arose de novo in all 5, and 4/5 had transient episodes of liver dysfunction in infancy. While a rare cause of NDM, the identification of *EIF2B1* heterozygous mutations in individuals with neonatal and early-onset diabetes is important to guide management of liver dysfunction in infancy to improve prognosis.

4.3.3.7 Neonatal and Early-Onset Diabetes Caused by Autosomal Recessive *YIPF5* Mutations

Homozygous mutations in the *YIPF5* gene have been recently reported to cause neonatal/early-onset diabetes with microcephaly and epilepsy in 6 individuals from 5 unrelated families [86]. All individuals were born small for gestational age and were diagnosed with diabetes between 4 weeks and 15 months. Individuals with this subtype of syndromic NDM have a phenotype almost identical to those with recessive mutations in *IER3IP1*, suggesting that these two genes may act in the same pathway. Functional studies suggested that the mutations identified in these families are unlikely to result in a complete loss of YIPF5 function, which may be incompatible with life.

4.3.4 Monogenic Autoimmune Beta-Cell Destruction

Approximately 2% of patients presenting with diabetes in the first 6 months of life have a mutation in a gene key for immune homeostasis. These patients may have normal birthweights but rapidly develop autoimmunity against beta-cells resulting in their complete loss and subsequent absence of insulin secretion. Around 50% of individuals have islet autoantibodies (GADA, IA2A, ZnT8A) [87]. The phenotype of these monogenic autoimmune syndromes is highly variable but usually patients develop additional autoimmunity against other endocrine organs (e.g., hypothyroidism), the gut (e.g., enteropathy), and autoimmune lymphoproliferative disorders. These may develop in infancy or can present later in life. Most patients require intense immunosuppressive treatment which may have limited efficacy, and hematopoietic stem cell transplantation is the only curative therapy. Once the beta-cells have been destroyed by autoimmunity and diabetes has developed, patients continue to require insulin therapy even after transplantation. Some patients can be successfully treated with targeted therapies specific to the genetic pathway affected (see below).

4.3.4.1 Neonatal and Early-Onset Diabetes Caused by X-Linked Recessive *FOXP3* Mutations

Hemizygous mutations in the *FOXP3* gene cause Immunodysregulation, Polyendocrinopathy, enteropathy, X-linked (IPEX) syndrome, which affects males (with female carriers being unaffected). This is the most common form of monogenic autoimmunity, with >195 cases reported to date [88]. Boys with IPEX syndrome typically present with autoimmune enteropathy (in >95% of cases) and go on to develop diabetes (~50%) and severe atopic dermatitis (~60%). Hematological disorders are also common (~40%) and patients often have recurrent severe infections which may be secondary to their enteropathy. Diabetes may present after the age of 6 months and may be the sole feature at genetic testing. FOXP3 is a transcription factor key for regulatory T cell (Treg) development and suppressive capacity, and its loss results in reduced Treg number and/or function [89]. Rapamycin (AKA sirolimus) is the optimal immunosuppressive treatment as it preferentially acts on effector T-cells while boosting the suppressive function of Tregs if present [90].

4.3.4.2 Neonatal Diabetes Caused by Autosomal Recessive *IL2RA* Mutations

Biallelic loss of function mutations in *IL2RA* (also known as CD25) cause immunodeficiency 41 with lymphoproliferation and autoimmunity [91]. NDM has been reported in 1/4 of published cases [92] and in 4 additional cases in the University of Exeter Molecular Genomics Laboratory (unpublished data). All 4 published cases had enteropathy, atopic dermatitis, and recurrent infections [93]. *IL2RA* encodes the interleukin-2 receptor alpha chain, a subunit of the high-affinity IL2 receptor present in T and B cells as well as other immune cells. This receptor is highly expressed on Tregs and is key for the induction of the expression of FOXP3 and subsequent differentiation of Tregs [94].

4.3.4.3 Neonatal Diabetes Caused by Autosomal Recessive *LRBA* Mutations

Biallelic loss of function mutations in *LRBA* cause common variable immunodeficiency 8 with autoimmunity (CDID-8) [95]. The most common feature of this disorder is enteropathy, seen in >60% of cases, with autoimmune hemolytic anemia and idiopathic thrombocytic purpura diagnosed in approximately half of the cases [96]. The autoimmune manifestations are often complicated by recurrent infections of the respiratory tract, largely due to a failure of the humoral immune response. Diabetes is seen in ~25% of cases, with at least 12 having NDM as the presenting feature [97]. LRBA co-localizes on intracellular vesicles with CTLA-4, a potent suppressive immune receptor molecule, and prevents lysosomal degradation of these vesicles [98] therefore maintaining immune cell stores of CTLA-4. In a landmark study in 2015, Lo et al. showed that individuals with biallelic *LRBA* mutations responded well to targeted treatment with abatacept, a CTLA-4 Immunoglobulin fusion drug that partially replaces the lost suppressive signaling in these individuals.

4.3.4.4 Neonatal Diabetes Caused by Autosomal Dominant *STAT3* Mutation

Germline heterozygous gain-of-function mutations in *STAT3* cause Autoimmune Disease, Multisystem, Infantile-Onset, 1 (ADMIO1). Diabetes is present in ~25% of cases, with a median age at onset of around 8 weeks [99]. In some individuals, NDM is the presenting and only feature at genetic testing [100]. Other features commonly diagnosed in these patients include autoimmune cytopenias (~60%), lymphoproliferation (~60%), and autoimmune enteropathy (~55%). Short stature is also common, with ~70% of individuals having restricted growth. STAT3 is a signal transducer and transcription factor that is key for the regulation of multiple cellular processes in response to extracellular stimuli, including cell proliferation, differentiation, and death by apoptosis. *STAT3* gain-of-function mutations act by increasing STAT3 signaling, either under non-stimulated conditions or increasing activity under stimulus by cytokines. STAT3 has a key role in the development of Tregs, and some patients show reduced Treg numbers [100–102]. Targeted therapy with tocilizumab (an anti-IL6 receptor monoclonal antibody) has been shown to be effective in 8/9 individuals in whom it was tried, reducing autoimmunity [99].

4.3.4.5 Neonatal Diabetes Caused by Trisomy 21

Trisomy 21 causes Down syndrome. Childhood-onset diabetes is four times more common in individuals with Down syndrome than in the general population. These individuals are more likely to have HLA risk alleles for diabetes (DR3 and/or DR4) than the general population but have around half the HLA risk of type 1 diabetes as a group [103]. This intermediate HLA risk profile suggests either trisomy 21 reduces the HLA load needed to develop type 1 diabetes in Down syndrome or could suggest a mixed population, with some individuals coincidentally developing HLA-mediated type 1 diabetes and others with non-HLA-mediated diabetes. It was recently shown that some individuals with Down syndrome presented with NDM and did not have higher levels of risk HLA alleles than the general population, making them unlikely to have coincidental Down syndrome and type 1 diabetes [104]. This subtype of NDM is thought to be autoimmune as patients often have islet autoantibodies and may develop additional autoimmunity, though further studies are needed to elucidate the underlying mechanism.

4.3.5 Early-Onset Type 1 Diabetes

While the vast majority of patients diagnosed with diabetes before 6 months have a monogenic aetiology, it was recently shown that ~4% have extreme early-onset type 1 diabetes [105]. These individuals have a rapid loss of beta-cells shown by very low or absent C-peptide within weeks of diagnosis and commonly have islet-autoantibodies (GADA, IA2A, and ZnT8A). There is evidence some of these individuals have reduced insulin secretion in utero, as many had low birthweight which correlated with age at presentation. A diagnosis of type 1 diabetes in patients with diabetes onset before the age of 6 months is by a negative finding upon comprehensive genetic testing of all known causes combined with a high type 1 diabetes genetic risk score [106]. Genetic testing, therefore, remains crucial for all individuals diagnosed before the age of 6 months.

4.3.6 6q24 Methylation Defects Causing Transient Neonatal Diabetes

Methylation defects resulting in overexpression of the differentially methylated genes at the 6q24 locus *PLAGL1* and *HYMAI* are a common cause of TNDM [107]. At this locus, methylation of maternally inherited alleles results in expression of the paternally inherited copy of the genes [108]. Three mechanisms are known to result in this TNDM subtype: paternal uniparental disomy (UPD), duplication of the paternal allele, and loss of methylation of the maternal allele [109].

Affected individuals have insulin deficiency in utero resulting in IUGR [3]. Their diabetes is generally diagnosed in the first hours of life and requires insulin treatment. Additional clinical features are sometimes present, including umbilical hernia, macroglossia and, rarely, neurological defects [109]. In patients with 6q24 methylation defects diabetes generally remits before 3 months of age but relapses later in life [107].

4.3.6.1 Transient Neonatal Diabetes Caused by Autosomal Recessive *ZFP57* Mutations

About 10% of patients with TNDM caused by a 6q24 methylation defect have a loss of methylation at multiple loci due to biallelic mutations in *ZFP57* [107, 110]. This transcription factor is essential to maintain parental imprinting. Individuals with loss of function mutations in *ZFP57* develop TNDM as a result of loss of maternal methylation at 6q24 and have a spectrum of extra-pancreatic features depending on the other parentally imprinted loci affected.

4.4 Conclusions

As more genetic causes of neonatal and early-onset diabetes are discovered, classification of the disease is increasingly relying on identifying the molecular defects causing the disease. The identification and characterization of over 30 genetic causes of NDM have shown that, while some genetic causes clearly map to a specific clinical subtype (for example, 6q24 TNDM), mutations in many aetiological genes result in a spectrum of diabetes, which sometimes overlaps all 3 clinical categories (for example, mutations in the potassium channel genes *ABCC8* and *KCNJ11*, which depending on the mutation can cause TNDM, PNDM, or DEND syndrome). This highlights the complexity of NDM and the challenges in interpreting genetic results and defining prognosis (Fig. 4.2).

Early, comprehensive testing for all known genetic causes of NDM is essential for the patients' clinical management and allows accurate classification of the clinical and genetic subtype before the patients have developed additional features or their diabetes has remitted [9]. This is essential to improve outcomes for patients

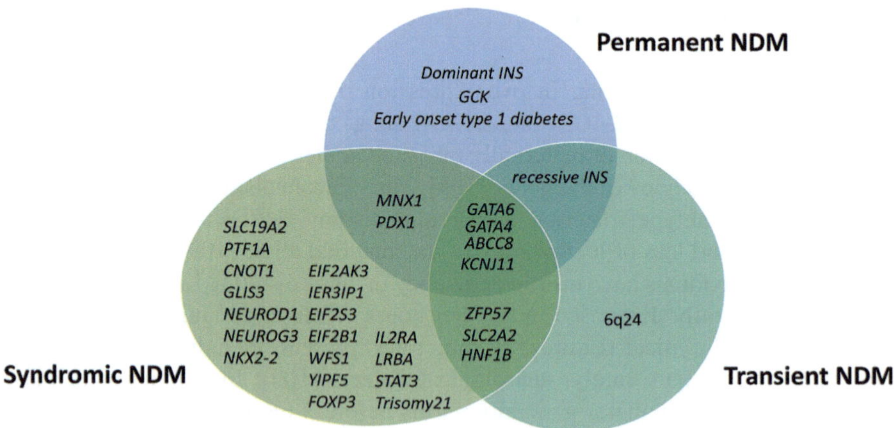

Fig. 4.2 Venn diagram of clinical and genetic classification of NDM

with neonatal and early-onset diabetes and is one successful example of the application of precision medicine to diagnosis and care of individuals with a rare genetic condition.

References

1. Edghill EL, Dix RJ, Flanagan SE, Bingley PJ, Hattersley AT, Ellard S, et al. HLA genotyping supports a nonautoimmune etiology in patients diagnosed with diabetes under the age of 6 months. Diabetes. 2006;55(6):1895–8.
2. Iafusco D, Stazi MA, Cotichini R, Cotellessa M, Martinucci ME, Mazzella M, et al. Permanent diabetes mellitus in the first year of life. Diabetologia. 2002;45(6):798–804.
3. Flanagan SE, Patch AM, Mackay DJ, Edghill EL, Gloyn AL, Robinson D, et al. Mutations in ATP-sensitive K+ channel genes cause transient neonatal diabetes and permanent diabetes in childhood or adulthood. Diabetes. 2007;56(7):1930–7.
4. Gardner RJ, Mackay DJ, Mungall AJ, Polychronakos C, Siebert R, Shield JP, et al. An imprinted locus associated with transient neonatal diabetes mellitus. Hum Mol Genet. 2000;9(4):589–96.
5. Babenko AP, Polak M, Cave H, Busiah K, Czernichow P, Scharfmann R, et al. Activating mutations in the ABCC8 gene in neonatal diabetes mellitus. N Engl J Med. 2006;355(5):456–66.
6. Gloyn AL, Reimann F, Girard C, Edghill EL, Proks P, Pearson ER, et al. Relapsing diabetes can result from moderately activating mutations in KCNJ11. Hum Mol Genet. 2005;14(7):925–34.
7. Pearson ER, Flechtner I, Njolstad PR, Malecki MT, Flanagan SE, Larkin B, et al. Switching from insulin to oral sulfonylureas in patients with diabetes due to Kir6.2 mutations. N Engl J Med. 2006;355(5):467–77.
8. Rafiq M, Flanagan SE, Patch AM, Shields BM, Ellard S, Hattersley AT. Effective treatment with oral sulfonylureas in patients with diabetes due to sulfonylurea receptor 1 (SUR1) mutations. Diabetes Care. 2008;31(2):204–9.
9. De Franco E, Flanagan SE, Houghton JA, Lango Allen H, Mackay DJ, Temple IK, et al. The effect of early, comprehensive genomic testing on clinical care in neonatal diabetes: an international cohort study. Lancet. 2015;386(9997):957–63.
10. Allen HL, Flanagan SE, Shaw-Smith C, De Franco E, Akerman I, Caswell R, et al. GATA6 haploinsufficiency causes pancreatic agenesis in humans. Nat Genet. 2011;44(1):20–2.
11. Gloyn AL, Pearson ER, Antcliff JF, Proks P, Bruining GJ, Slingerland AS, et al. Activating mutations in the gene encoding the ATP-sensitive potassium-channel subunit Kir6.2 and permanent neonatal diabetes. N Engl J Med. 2004;350(18):1838–49.
12. Proks P, Arnold AL, Bruining J, Girard C, Flanagan SE, Larkin B, et al. A heterozygous activating mutation in the sulphonylurea receptor SUR1 (ABCC8) causes neonatal diabetes. Hum Mol Genet. 2006;15(11):1793–800.
13. Ellard S, Flanagan SE, Girard CA, Patch AM, Harries LW, Parrish A, et al. Permanent neonatal diabetes caused by dominant, recessive, or compound heterozygous SUR1 mutations with opposite functional effects. Am J Hum Genet. 2007;81(2):375–82.
14. Bowman P, Day J, Torrens L, Shepherd MH, Knight BA, Ford TJ, et al. Cognitive, neurological, and behavioral features in adults with KCNJ11 neonatal diabetes. Diabetes Care. 2019;42(2):215–24.
15. Busiah K, Drunat S, Vaivre-Douret L, Bonnefond A, Simon A, Flechtner I, et al. Neuropsychological dysfunction and developmental defects associated with genetic changes in infants with neonatal diabetes mellitus: a prospective cohort study [corrected]. Lancet Diabetes Endocrinol. 2013;1(3):199–207.

16. Bowman P, Sulen A, Barbetti F, Beltrand J, Svalastoga P, Codner E, et al. Effectiveness and safety of long-term treatment with sulfonylureas in patients with neonatal diabetes due to KCNJ11 mutations: an international cohort study. Lancet Diabetes Endocrinol. 2018;6:637.
17. Bowman P, Mathews F, Barbetti F, Shepherd MH, Sanchez J, Piccini B, et al. Long-term follow-up of glycemic and neurological outcomes in an international series of patients with sulfonylurea-treated ABCC8 permanent neonatal diabetes. Diabetes Care. 2021;44(1):35–42.
18. Garin I, Edghill EL, Akerman I, Rubio-Cabezas O, Rica I, Locke JM, et al. Recessive mutations in the INS gene result in neonatal diabetes through reduced insulin biosynthesis. Proc Natl Acad Sci U S A. 2010;107(7):3105–10.
19. Njolstad PR, Sovik O, Cuesta-Munoz A, Bjorkhaug L, Massa O, Barbetti F, et al. Neonatal diabetes mellitus due to complete glucokinase deficiency. N Engl J Med. 2001;344(21):1588–92.
20. Vionnet N, Stoffel M, Takeda J, Yasuda K, Bell GI, Zouali H, et al. Nonsense mutation in the glucokinase gene causes early-onset non-insulin-dependent diabetes mellitus. Nature. 1992;356(6371):721–2.
21. Raimondo A, Chakera AJ, Thomsen SK, Colclough K, Barrett A, De Franco E, et al. Phenotypic severity of homozygous GCK mutations causing neonatal or childhood-onset diabetes is primarily mediated through effects on protein stability. Hum Mol Genet. 2014;23(24):6432–40.
22. Santer R, Groth S, Kinner M, Dombrowski A, Berry GT, Brodehl J, et al. The mutation spectrum of the facilitative glucose transporter gene SLC2A2 (GLUT2) in patients with Fanconi-Bickel syndrome. Hum Genet. 2002;110(1):21–9.
23. Sansbury FH, Flanagan SE, Houghton JA, Shuixian Shen FL, Al-Senani AM, Habeb AM, et al. SLC2A2 mutations can cause neonatal diabetes, suggesting GLUT2 may have a role in human insulin secretion. Diabetologia. 2012;55(9):2381–5.
24. Labay V, Raz T, Baron D, Mandel H, Williams H, Barrett T, et al. Mutations in SLC19A2 cause thiamine-responsive megaloblastic anaemia associated with diabetes mellitus and deafness. Nat Genet. 1999;22(3):300–4.
25. Bay A, Keskin M, Hizli S, Uygun H, Dai A, Gumruk F. Thiamine-responsive megaloblastic anemia syndrome. Int J Hematol. 2010;92(3):524–6.
26. Bergmann AK, Sahai I, Falcone JF, Fleming J, Bagg A, Borgna-Pignati C, et al. Thiamine-responsive megaloblastic anemia: identification of novel compound heterozygotes and mutation update. J Pediatr. 2009;155(6):888–92.e1.
27. Mandel H, Berant M, Hazani A, Naveh Y. Thiamine-dependent beriberi in the "thiamine-responsive anemia syndrome". N Engl J Med. 1984;311(13):836–8.
28. Habeb AM, Flanagan SE, Zulali MA, Abdullah MA, Pomahacova R, Boyadzhiev V, et al. Pharmacogenomics in diabetes: outcomes of thiamine therapy in TRMA syndrome. Diabetologia. 2018;61(5):1027–36.
29. De Franco E, Watson RA, Weninger WJ, Wong CC, Flanagan SE, Caswell R, et al. A specific CNOT1 mutation results in a novel syndrome of pancreatic agenesis and holoprosencephaly through impaired pancreatic and neurological development. Am J Hum Genet. 2019;104(5):985–9.
30. Stoffers DA, Zinkin NT, Stanojevic V, Clarke WL, Habener JF. Pancreatic agenesis attributable to a single nucleotide deletion in the human IPF1 gene coding sequence. Nat Genet. 1997;15(1):106–10.
31. Jonsson J, Carlsson L, Edlund T, Edlund H. Insulin-promoter-factor 1 is required for pancreas development in mice. Nature. 1994;371(6498):606–9.
32. Nicolino M, Claiborn KC, Senee V, Boland A, Stoffers DA, Julier C. A novel hypomorphic PDX1 mutation responsible for permanent neonatal diabetes with subclinical exocrine deficiency. Diabetes. 2010;59(3):733–40.
33. De Franco E, Shaw-Smith C, Flanagan SE, Edghill EL, Wolf J, Otte V, et al. Biallelic PDX1 (insulin promoter factor 1) mutations causing neonatal diabetes without exocrine pancreatic insufficiency. Diabet Med. 2013;30(5):e197–200.

34. Sellick GS, Barker KT, Stolte-Dijkstra I, Fleischmann C, Coleman RJ, Garrett C, et al. Mutations in PTF1A cause pancreatic and cerebellar agenesis. Nat Genet. 2004;36(12):1301–5.
35. Weedon MN, Cebola I, Patch AM, Flanagan SE, De Franco E, Caswell R, et al. Recessive mutations in a distal PTF1A enhancer cause isolated pancreatic agenesis. Nat Genet. 2014;46(1):61–4.
36. Demirbilek H, Cayir A, Flanagan SE, Yıldırım R, Kor Y, Gurbuz F, et al. Clinical characteristics and long-term follow-up of patients with diabetes due to PTF1A enhancer mutations. J Clin Endocrinol Metab. 2020;105(12):e4351–9.
37. Houghton JA, Swift GH, Shaw-Smith C, Flanagan SE, de Franco E, Caswell R, et al. Isolated pancreatic aplasia due to a hypomorphic PTF1A mutation. Diabetes. 2016;65(9):2810–5.
38. Horikawa Y, Iwasaki N, Hara M, Furuta H, Hinokio Y, Cockburn BN, et al. Mutation in hepatocyte nuclear factor-1 beta gene (TCF2) associated with MODY. Nat Genet. 1997;17(4):384–5.
39. Bellanne-Chantelot C, Chauveau D, Gautier JF, Dubois-Laforgue D, Clauin S, Beaufils S, et al. Clinical spectrum associated with hepatocyte nuclear factor-1beta mutations. Ann Intern Med. 2004;140(7):510–7.
40. Yorifuji T, Kurokawa K, Mamada M, Imai T, Kawai M, Nishi Y, et al. Neonatal diabetes mellitus and neonatal polycystic, dysplastic kidneys: phenotypically discordant recurrence of a mutation in the hepatocyte nuclear factor-1beta gene due to germline mosaicism. J Clin Endocrinol Metab. 2004;89(6):2905–8.
41. Edghill EL, Bingham C, Slingerland AS, Minton JA, Noordam C, Ellard S, et al. Hepatocyte nuclear factor-1 beta mutations cause neonatal diabetes and intrauterine growth retardation: support for a critical role of HNF-1beta in human pancreatic development. Diabet Med. 2006;23(12):1301–6.
42. Smith SB, Qu HQ, Taleb N, Kishimoto NY, Scheel DW, Lu Y, et al. Rfx6 directs islet formation and insulin production in mice and humans. Nature. 2010;463(7282):775–80.
43. Sansbury FH, Kirel B, Caswell R, Lango Allen H, Flanagan SE, Hattersley AT, et al. Biallelic RFX6 mutations can cause childhood as well as neonatal onset diabetes mellitus. Eur J Hum Genet. 2015;23:1750.
44. Spiegel R, Dobbie A, Hartman C, de Vries L, Ellard S, Shalev SA. Clinical characterization of a newly described neonatal diabetes syndrome caused by RFX6 mutations. Am J Med Genet A. 2011;155a(11):2821–5.
45. Patel KA, Kettunen J, Laakso M, Stancakova A, Laver TW, Colclough K, et al. Heterozygous RFX6 protein truncating variants are associated with MODY with reduced penetrance. Nat Commun. 2017;8(1):888.
46. Kodo K, Nishizawa T, Furutani M, Arai S, Yamamura E, Joo K, et al. GATA6 mutations cause human cardiac outflow tract defects by disrupting semaphorin-plexin signaling. Proc Natl Acad Sci U S A. 2009;106(33):13933–8.
47. De Franco E, Shaw-Smith C, Flanagan SE, Shepherd MH, Hattersley AT, Ellard S. GATA6 mutations cause a broad phenotypic spectrum of diabetes from pancreatic agenesis to adult-onset diabetes without exocrine insufficiency. Diabetes. 2013;62(3):993–7.
48. Rajagopal SK, Ma Q, Obler D, Shen J, Manichaikul A, Tomita-Mitchell A, et al. Spectrum of heart disease associated with murine and human GATA4 mutation. J Mol Cell Cardiol. 2007;43(6):677–85.
49. Tomita-Mitchell A, Maslen CL, Morris CD, Garg V, Goldmuntz E. GATA4 sequence variants in patients with congenital heart disease. J Med Genet. 2007;44(12):779–83.
50. D'Amato E, Giacopelli F, Giannattasio A, D'Annunzio G, Bocciardi R, Musso M, et al. Genetic investigation in an Italian child with an unusual association of atrial septal defect, attributable to a new familial GATA4 gene mutation, and neonatal diabetes due to pancreatic agenesis. Diabet Med. 2010;27(10):1195–200.
51. Shaw-Smith C, De Franco E, Lango Allen H, Batlle M, Flanagan SE, Borowiec M, et al. GATA4 mutations are a cause of neonatal and childhood-onset diabetes. Diabetes. 2014;63(8):2888–94.

52. Kruszka P, Berger SI, Weiss K, Everson JL, Martinez AF, Hong S, et al. A CCR4-NOT transcription complex, subunit 1, CNOT1, variant associated with Holoprosencephaly. Am J Hum Genet. 2019;104(5):990–3.
53. Senee V, Chelala C, Duchatelet S, Feng D, Blanc H, Cossec JC, et al. Mutations in GLIS3 are responsible for a rare syndrome with neonatal diabetes mellitus and congenital hypothyroidism. Nat Genet. 2006;38:682–7.
54. Alghamdi KA, Alsaedi AB, Aljasser A, Altawil A, Kamal NM. Extended clinical features associated with novel Glis3 mutation: a case report. BMC Endocr Disord. 2017;17(1):14.
55. Dimitri P, De Franco E, Habeb AM, Gurbuz F, Moussa K, Taha D, et al. An emerging, recognizable facial phenotype in association with mutations in GLI-similar 3 (GLIS3). Am J Med Genet A. 2016;170(7):1918–23.
56. Splittstoesser V, Vollbach H, Plamper M, Garbe W, De Franco E, Houghton JAL, et al. Case report: extended clinical spectrum of the neonatal diabetes with congenital hypothyroidism syndrome. Front Endocrinol (Lausanne). 2021;12:665336.
57. Dimitri P, Habeb AM, Gurbuz F, Millward A, Wallis S, Moussa K, et al. Expanding the clinical spectrum associated with GLIS3 mutations. J Clin Endocrinol Metab. 2015;100(10):E1362–9.
58. Demirbilek H, Hatipoglu N, Gul U, Tatli ZU, Ellard S, Flanagan SE, et al. Permanent neonatal diabetes mellitus and neurological abnormalities due to a novel homozygous missense mutation in NEUROD1. Pediatr Diabetes. 2018;19:898.
59. Rubio-Cabezas O, Minton JA, Kantor I, Williams D, Ellard S, Hattersley AT. Homozygous mutations in NEUROD1 are responsible for a novel syndrome of permanent neonatal diabetes and neurological abnormalities. Diabetes. 2010;59(9):2326–31.
60. Wang J, Cortina G, Wu SV, Tran R, Cho JH, Tsai MJ, et al. Mutant neurogenin-3 in congenital malabsorptive diarrhea. N Engl J Med. 2006;355(3):270–80.
61. Hancili S, Bonnefond A, Philippe J, Vaillant E, De Graeve F, Sand O, et al. A novel NEUROG3 mutation in neonatal diabetes associated with a neuro-intestinal syndrome. Pediatr Diabetes. 2018;19(3):381–7.
62. Pinney SE, Oliver-Krasinski J, Ernst L, Hughes N, Patel P, Stoffers DA, et al. Neonatal diabetes and congenital malabsorptive diarrhea attributable to a novel mutation in the human neurogenin-3 gene coding sequence. J Clin Endocrinol Metab. 2011;96(7):1960–5.
63. Rubio-Cabezas O, Jensen JN, Hodgson MI, Codner E, Ellard S, Serup P, et al. Permanent neonatal diabetes and enteric anendocrinosis associated with biallelic mutations in NEUROG3. Diabetes. 2011;60(4):1349–53.
64. Solorzano-Vargas RS, Bjerknes M, Wang J, Wu SV, Garcia-Careaga MG, Pitukcheewanont P, et al. Null mutations of NEUROG3 are associated with delayed-onset diabetes mellitus. JCI Insight. 2020;5(1)
65. Auerbach A, Cohen A, Ofek Shlomai N, Weinberg-Shukron A, Gulsuner S, King MC, et al. NKX2-2 mutation causes congenital diabetes and infantile obesity with paradoxical glucose-induced ghrelin secretion. J Clin Endocrinol Metab. 2020;105(11):3486.
66. Flanagan SE, De Franco E, Lango Allen H, Zerah M, Abdul-Rasoul MM, Edge JA, et al. Analysis of transcription factors key for mouse pancreatic development establishes NKX2-2 and MNX1 mutations as causes of neonatal diabetes in man. Cell Metab. 2014;19(1):146–54.
67. Ross AJ, Ruiz-Perez V, Wang Y, Hagan DM, Scherer S, Lynch SA, et al. A homeobox gene, HLXB9, is the major locus for dominantly inherited sacral agenesis. Nat Genet. 1998;20(4):358–61.
68. Bonnefond A, Vaillant E, Philippe J, Skrobek B, Lobbens S, Yengo L, et al. Transcription factor gene MNX1 is a novel cause of permanent neonatal diabetes in a consanguineous family. Diabetes Metab. 2013;39(3):276–80.
69. Stoy J, Edghill EL, Flanagan SE, Ye H, Paz VP, Pluzhnikov A, et al. Insulin gene mutations as a cause of permanent neonatal diabetes. Proc Natl Acad Sci U S A. 2007;104(38):15040–4.
70. Delepine M, Nicolino M, Barrett T, Golamaully M, Lathrop GM, Julier C. EIF2AK3, encoding translation initiation factor 2-alpha kinase 3, is mutated in patients with Wolcott-Rallison syndrome. Nat Genet. 2000;25(4):406–9.

71. Rubio-Cabezas O, Patch AM, Minton JA, Flanagan SE, Edghill EL, Hussain K, et al. Wolcott-Rallison syndrome is the most common genetic cause of permanent neonatal diabetes in consanguineous families. J Clin Endocrinol Metab. 2009;94(11):4162–70.
72. Julier C, Nicolino M. Wolcott-Rallison syndrome. Orphanet J Rare Dis. 2010;5:29.
73. Deeb A, Habeb A, Kaplan W, Attia S, Hadi S, Osman A, et al. Genetic characteristics, clinical spectrum, and incidence of neonatal diabetes in the emirate of Abu Dhabi, United Arab Emirates. Am J Med Genet A. 2016;170(3):602–9.
74. Nordström J, Lundgren M, Jorns C, Fischler B, Arnell H, Dlugosz R, et al. First European case of simultaneous liver and pancreas transplantation as treatment of Wolcott-Rallison syndrome in a small child. Transplantation. 2020;104(3):522–5.
75. Rivera E, Gupta S, Chavers B, Quinones L, Berger MR, Schwarzenberg SJ, et al. En bloc multiorgan transplant (liver, pancreas, and kidney) for acute liver and renal failure in a patient with Wolcott-Rallison syndrome. Liver Transpl. 2016;22(3):371–4.
76. Tzakis AG, Nunnelley MJ, Tekin A, Buccini LD, Garcia J, Uchida K, et al. Liver, pancreas and kidney transplantation for the treatment of Wolcott-Rallison syndrome. Am J Transplant. 2015;15(2):565–7.
77. Poulton CJ, Schot R, Kia SK, Jones M, Verheijen FW, Venselaar H, et al. Microcephaly with simplified gyration, epilepsy, and infantile diabetes linked to inappropriate apoptosis of neural progenitors. Am J Hum Genet. 2011;89(2):265–76.
78. Abdel-Salam GM, Schaffer AE, Zaki MS, Dixon-Salazar T, Mostafa IS, Afifi HH, et al. A homozygous IER3IP1 mutation causes microcephaly with simplified gyral pattern, epilepsy, and permanent neonatal diabetes syndrome (MEDS). Am J Med Genet A. 2012;158a(11):2788–96.
79. Shalev SA, Tenenbaum-Rakover Y, Horovitz Y, Paz VP, Ye H, Carmody D, et al. Microcephaly, epilepsy, and neonatal diabetes due to compound heterozygous mutations in IER3IP1: insights into the natural history of a rare disorder. Pediatr Diabetes. 2014;15(3):252–6.
80. Valenzuela I, Boronat S, Martínez-Sáez E, Clemente M, Sánchez-Montañez Á, Munell F, et al. Microcephaly with simplified gyral pattern, epilepsy and permanent neonatal diabetes syndrome (MEDS). A new patient and review of the literature. Eur J Med Genet. 2017;60(10):517–20.
81. Skopkova M, Hennig F, Shin BS, Turner CE, Stanikova D, Brennerova K, et al. EIF2S3 mutations associated with severe X-linked intellectual disability syndrome MEHMO. Hum Mutat. 2017;38(4):409–25.
82. de Heredia ML, Clèries R, Nunes V. Genotypic classification of patients with Wolfram syndrome: insights into the natural history of the disease and correlation with phenotype. Genet Med. 2013;15(7):497–506.
83. De Franco E, Flanagan SE, Yagi T, Abreu D, Mahadevan J, Johnson MB, et al. Dominant ER stress-inducing WFS1 mutations underlie a genetic syndrome of neonatal/infancy-onset diabetes, congenital sensorineural deafness, and congenital cataracts. Diabetes. 2017;66(7):2044–53.
84. van der Knaap MS, Leegwater PA, Konst AA, Visser A, Naidu S, Oudejans CB, et al. Mutations in each of the five subunits of translation initiation factor eIF2B can cause leukoencephalopathy with vanishing white matter. Ann Neurol. 2002;51(2):264–70.
85. De Franco E, Caswell R, Johnson MB, Wakeling MN, Zung A, Dung VC, et al. De novo mutations in EIF2B1 affecting eIF2 signaling cause neonatal/early onset diabetes and transient hepatic dysfunction. Diabetes. 2019.
86. De Franco E, Lytrivi M, Ibrahim H, Montaser H, Wakeling MN, Fantuzzi F, et al. YIPF5 mutations cause neonatal diabetes and microcephaly through endoplasmic reticulum stress. J Clin Invest. 2020;130(12):6338–53.
87. Johnson MB, Patel KA, De Franco E, Houghton JAL, McDonald TJ, Ellard S, et al. A type 1 diabetes genetic risk score can discriminate monogenic autoimmunity with diabetes from early-onset clustering of polygenic autoimmunity with diabetes. Diabetologia. 2018;61(4):862–9.

88. Park JH, Lee KH, Jeon B, Ochs HD, Lee JS, Gee HY, et al. Immune dysregulation, polyendocrinopathy, enteropathy, X-linked (IPEX) syndrome: a systematic review. Autoimmun Rev. 2020;19(6):102526.
89. Fontenot JD, Gavin MA, Rudensky AY. Foxp3 programs the development and function of CD4+CD25+ regulatory T cells. Nat Immunol. 2003;4(4):330–6.
90. Passerini L, Barzaghi F, Curto R, Sartirana C, Barera G, Tucci F, et al. Treatment with rapamycin can restore regulatory T-cell function in IPEX patients. J Allergy Clin Immunol. 2020;145(4):1262–71.e13.
91. Sharfe N, Dadi HK, Shahar M, Roifman CM. Human immune disorder arising from mutation of the alpha chain of the interleukin-2 receptor. Proc Natl Acad Sci U S A. 1997;94(7):3168–71.
92. Caudy AA, Reddy ST, Chatila T, Atkinson JP, Verbsky JW. CD25 deficiency causes an immune dysregulation, polyendocrinopathy, enteropathy, X-linked-like syndrome, and defective IL-10 expression from CD4 lymphocytes. J Allergy Clin Immunol. 2007;119(2):482–7.
93. Johnson MB, Hattersley AT, Flanagan SE. Monogenic autoimmune diseases of the endocrine system. Lancet Diabetes Endocrinol. 2016;4(10):862–72.
94. Zorn E, Nelson EA, Mohseni M, Porcheray F, Kim H, Litsa D, et al. IL-2 regulates FOXP3 expression in human CD4+CD25+ regulatory T cells through a STAT-dependent mechanism and induces the expansion of these cells in vivo. Blood. 2006;108(5):1571–9.
95. Lopez-Herrera G, Tampella G, Pan-Hammarstrom Q, Herholz P, Trujillo-Vargas CM, Phadwal K, et al. Deleterious mutations in LRBA are associated with a syndrome of immune deficiency and autoimmunity. Am J Hum Genet. 2012;90(6):986–1001.
96. Habibi S, Zaki-Dizaji M, Rafiemanesh H, Lo B, Jamee M, Gámez-Díaz L, et al. Clinical, immunologic, and molecular spectrum of patients with LPS-responsive beige-like anchor protein deficiency: a systematic review. J Allergy Clin Immunol Pract. 2019;7(7):2379–86.e5.
97. Johnson MB, De Franco E, Lango Allen H, Al Senani A, Elbarbary N, Siklar Z, et al. Recessively inherited LRBA mutations cause autoimmunity presenting as neonatal diabetes. Diabetes. 2017;66(8):2316–22.
98. Lo B, Zhang K, Lu W, Zheng L, Zhang Q, Kanellopoulou C, et al. AUTOIMMUNE DISEASE. Patients with LRBA deficiency show CTLA4 loss and immune dysregulation responsive to abatacept therapy. Science. 2015;349(6246):436–40.
99. Fabre A, Marchal S, Barlogis V, Mari B, Barbry P, Rohrlich PS, et al. Clinical aspects of STAT3 gain-of-function germline mutations: a systematic review. J Allergy Clin Immunol Pract. 2019;7(6):1958–69.e9.
100. Flanagan SE, Haapaniemi E, Russell MA, Caswell R, Allen HL, De Franco E, et al. Activating germline mutations in STAT3 cause early-onset multi-organ autoimmune disease. Nat Genet. 2014;46(8):812–4.
101. Haapaniemi EM, Kaustio M, Rajala HL, van Adrichem AJ, Kainulainen L, Glumoff V, et al. Autoimmunity, hypogammaglobulinemia, lymphoproliferation, and mycobacterial disease in patients with activating mutations in STAT3. Blood. 2015;125(4):639–48.
102. Milner JD, Vogel TP, Forbes L, Ma CA, Stray-Pedersen A, Niemela JE, et al. Early-onset lymphoproliferation and autoimmunity caused by germline STAT3 gain-of-function mutations. Blood. 2015;125(4):591–9.
103. Aitken RJ, Mehers KL, Williams AJ, Brown J, Bingley PJ, Holl RW, et al. Early-onset, coexisting autoimmunity and decreased HLA-mediated susceptibility are the characteristics of diabetes in down syndrome. Diabetes Care. 2013;36(5):1181–5.
104. Johnson MB, De Franco E, Greeley SAW, Letourneau LR, Gillespie KM, Wakeling MN, et al. Trisomy 21 is a cause of permanent neonatal diabetes that is autoimmune but not HLA associated. Diabetes. 2019;68(7):1528–35.
105. Johnson MB, Patel KA, De Franco E, Hagopian W, Killian M, McDonald TJ, et al. Type 1 diabetes can present before the age of 6 months and is characterised by autoimmunity and rapid loss of beta cells. Diabetologia. 2020;63(12):2605–15.

106. Patel KA, Oram RA, Flanagan SE, De Franco E, Colclough K, Shepherd M, et al. Type 1 diabetes genetic risk score: a novel tool to discriminate monogenic and type 1 diabetes. Diabetes. 2016;65(7):2094–9.
107. Mackay DJ, Temple IK. Transient neonatal diabetes mellitus type 1. Am J Med Genet C Semin Med Genet. 2010;154c(3):335–42.
108. Temple IK, Gardner RJ, Robinson DO, Kibirige MS, Ferguson AW, Baum JD, et al. Further evidence for an imprinted gene for neonatal diabetes localised to chromosome 6q22-q23. Hum Mol Genet. 1996;5(8):1117–21.
109. Temple IK, Shield JP. Transient neonatal diabetes, a disorder of imprinting. J Med Genet. 2002;39(12):872–5.
110. Mackay DJ, Callaway JL, Marks SM, White HE, Acerini CL, Boonen SE, et al. Hypomethylation of multiple imprinted loci in individuals with transient neonatal diabetes is associated with mutations in ZFP57. Nat Genet. 2008;40(8):949–51.

Chapter 5
Rare Forms of Early Onset Diabetes

Ivana Rabbone, Valentino Cherubini, Adriana Franzese, Enza Mozzillo, Valentina Tiberi, Davide Tinti, Marina Tripodi, Angela Zanfardino, Alessia Piscopo, and Dario Iafusco

5.1 Introduction

Neonatal Diabetes Mellitus (NDM) is a rare disorder, predominantly monogenic in origin. Generally, NDM presents as persistent hyperglycemia within the first 6 months of life. Mutations involving the KCNJ11, ABCC8, and INS genes account for nearly 70% of monogenic causes of permanent neonatal diabetes mellitus. However, other monogenic mutations characterize rarer forms of neonatal diabetes [1, 2]. The following rare cases of NDM represent the extreme variability and uniqueness of the presentation of monogenic diabetes.

Supplementary Information The online version contains supplementary material available at https://doi.org/10.1007/978-3-031-07008-2_5.

I. Rabbone (✉)
Division of Pediatrics, Department of Health Sciences, University of Piemonte Orientale, Novara, Italy
e-mail: ivana.rabbone@uniupo.it

V. Cherubini · V. Tiberi
Department of Women's and Children's Health "G. Salesi Hospital", University of Ancona, Ancona, Italy

A. Franzese · E. Mozzillo · M. Tripodi
Department of Translational Medical Sciences, Sector of Pediatrics, University Federico II, Naples, Italy

D. Tinti
Department of Pediatrics, University of Turin, Turin, Italy

A. Zanfardino · A. Piscopo · D. Iafusco
Department of Woman, Child and General and Specialistic Surgery, University of Campania "Luigi Vanvitelli", Naples, Italy

I. Rabbone, D. Iafusco (eds.), *Neonatal and Early Onset Diabetes Mellitus*,
https://doi.org/10.1007/978-3-031-07008-2_5

5.1.1 *Case #1*

An 8-day-old newborn was admitted to the Neonatal Intensive Care Unit (NICU) in a cachectic state with repeated vomiting, severe dehydration (time refill>3 s), weight loss of 16.8% compared to neonatal weight, reduced spontaneous motility, and diffuse hypotonia. There was a family history of multiple abortions with the father homozygous for Methylenetetrahydrofolate reductase (MTHFR) mutation, mother heterozygous for MTHFR mutation. His sister was suffering from congenital immunodeficiency, CD25 deficiency, from Interleukin-2 Receptor Alpha (IL2RA) gene mutation (diagnosis made during pregnancy of the patient). Born at 38 + 6 weeks of gestation from programmed cesarean section after a normal pregnancy, adequate for gestational age, Apgar 9-10-10.

From the tests performed in NICU aimed at excluding infection or metabolic disease, hyperglycemia (first glycemic value 1505 mg/dl–83.56 mmol/L) with metabolic acidosis and ketonuria was highlighted, thus indicating neonatal diabetes. IV rehydration was immediately initiated, which was then associated with IV insulin therapy up to the maximum dosage of 0.1 U/kg/h due to the difficulty in obtaining effective glycemic control. In consideration of the family history, the patient was investigated for the mutation of the IL2RA gene, with evidence of IPEX-like syndrome due to CD25 deficiency. The genetic investigation revealed unknown parental consanguinity.

The clinical course of the newborn in NICU was complicated by the onset of seizures associated with EEG signs of diffuse brain distress for which phenobarbital boluses were performed and, in suspicion of cerebral edema, therapy with mannitol. Due to the deterioration of the general conditions, the baby was kept intubated and sedated for about 36 h, after which there was a gradual slow improvement of the general conditions.

The blood glucose values gradually normalized during the hospitalization and returned to the range 80–120 mg/dl (4.44–6.67 mmol/L).

At discharge, the insulin intake of 0.03 UI/kg/h allowed to keep the patient in euglycemia (considering a glucose intake of 13 g/kg/day all per os 180 ml/kg/day, 119 Kcal/kg/day).

Blood glucose sensor with a pump placed at 2 months of life.

Performed at 4 months of life, in another hospital, allogeneic hematopoietic stem cell (HSC) transplant. Before the transplant, the patient had a good glycemic and metabolic balance.

The following complications occurred post-transplant during hospitalization:

- Difficult glycemic control, with the need to stop using the pump and start IV insulin therapy. Subcutaneous insulin with pump system restarted after 2 months from HSC transplant.
- Graft versus host disease (GvHD) grade III total (intestinal G4, liver 0, skin 1) treated with steroid and mycophenolate mofetil.
- Echocardiographic findings of moderate left ventricle eccentric hypertrophy associated with periorbital edema, episodes of desaturation, hypertensive crisis, and pro-BNP elevation for which he needed antihypertensive therapy.

- Pseudomonas Putida carbapenemase-producing sepsis and blood culture positivity for *S. Hominis* and *Strenotrophomonas*, for which targeted multiple antibiotic therapies were performed.
- Reduced tolerance to cyclosporine, expressed with renal toxicity.

Tested at 1-year-old serum autoantibodies typical of T1D (ICA: positive, GAD65: positive, IA-2A: negative, IAA: negative).

IPEX Syndrome is a heritable autoimmune lymphoproliferative disease caused by loss of function mutation in FOXP3 [3] which maps to the X chromosome. The common phenotype found in classic IPEX is neonatal-onset insulin-dependent diabetes mellitus and an autoimmune enteropathy [4].

Several gene defects that affect T regulatory cell function give rise to IPEX-related phenotypes.

Human IL2RA null mutation, resulting in CD25 deficiency, results in an IPEX-like syndrome [5, 6]. While in IPEX Syndrome, Type 1 diabetes (T1D) is a frequent symptom, there are only three cases reported in the literature of patients with IPEX-like syndrome due to CD25 deficiency and T1D.

The case reported by Caudy et al. [6] developed at 6 weeks of age, severe diarrhea and insulin-dependent diabetes mellitus. Barzaghi et al. described two patients with CD25 mutation in their series, but only one had T1D with onset at 20 days of age [7]. The last reported case presented the onset of the disease at 5 months of age [8]. The onset of our patient at 8 days of life is the earliest reported in the literature.

5.1.2 Case #2

A male newborn came to our attention for persistent hyperglycemia a few hours after birth in June 2016.

He was born in a peripheral labor ward after 38 + 5 weeks of gestation, characterized by gestational diabetes treated with insulin. A familiar history (paternal, 2° line) of type 2 diabetes was present. During pregnancy, a growth below the 3rd centile was evident, and the child was born 2000 g (small for gestational age, SGA), with a length of 45 cm, and head circumference of 32 cm (all below 3rd centile). Neonatal cerebral and cardiac ultrasounds were normal.

During the first day of life, hyperglycemia was evident, which persisted in the following days and required a transferal in our center on the fourth day of life to initiate insulin therapy. The initial insulin dose was 0.01 UI/kg/day, given IV and then subcutaneously through an insulin pump. C-peptide at day 7 resulted in <0.3 ng/mL (normal value 1.10–4.40) and insulin, despite external supplementation, was lower than normal (0.5 microUI/mL). Antibodies testing resulted positive for 1 antibody (ICA, title 1:20, normal value <5). After a few days of blood glucose, continuous glucose monitoring (Dexcom G4, San Diego, USA) was initiated to better understand glucose fluctuations and to adjust insulin therapy accordingly. Pump and sensor placement was complicated, since skin resulted in dystrophic with eczematous dermatitis, with some episodes of folliculitis treated with topic antibiotics. Insulin was used diluted 1:10 (5 ml in 50 ml of specific insulin diluent) [9].

From 1 month of life, the child necessitated multiple erythropoietin injections, iron, B12, and folic acid supplementation for persistent anemia. Also, hypereosinophilia was noted (2540 eosinophils/mcL) with a high value of IgE (101 kUI/L), while IgA and IgM resulted within the normal range. Lymphocyte subpopulations resulted normal for age; thyroiditis and celiac screening was normal.

At the same time, persistent diarrhea developed, with positive Rotavirus antigen in stool. Chemical stool analysis showed steatorrhea, while other values, eosinophils as well as hemoglobin resulted normal. Serological milk-specific IgE resulted positive (1.6 kUA/L), therefore we changed preterm formula milk with hydrolyzed milk, with symptom persistence and a drop in weight gain. Gastric and duodenal mucosa showed signs of moderate chronic gastritis with duodenal villous flattening and lymphocyte infiltration. In the suspect of autoimmune enteritis, we performed anti-villin and anti-harmonin searches, which returned positive. Parenteral total nutrition was then started with IV insulin infusion.

In the suspect of Immunodysregulation Polyendocrinopathy Enteropathy X-linked (IPEX), we performed a genetic test on a blood sample, which resulted in a mutation on FOXP3 gene (c.736-1G > A), previously described in one patient [10] At 3 months of age, the child started immunosuppressive therapy with sirolimus and methylprednisolone, with good clinical result [11]. At 6 months of age, he underwent hematopoietic stem cell transplantation (HSCT). Unfortunately, the child died 1 week after the HSCT for an unknown cause (cardiac arrest).

5.1.3 Case #3

A son of consanguineous Hispanic parents (first cousins), delivered at 37 weeks of gestation with a weight of 1800 g was adopted at the age of 6 months. He was diagnosed with neonatal diabetes on the fifth day of life with fasting plasma glucose of 15.9 mmol/L (286 mg/dL) and undetectable serum C-peptide.

Placed on intravenous insulin therapy (0.05 IU/kg /hr), with substantial improvement of glucose levels within 9 days from treatment start. The subject was negative for autoantibodies in serum (i.e., ICA, GAD65, IA-2A, and IAA) typical of T1D at diagnosis of diabetes. Autoantibody assays were repeated throughout the first 3 years of life to confirm the patient did not have an immune-mediated form of diabetes. Moreover, antibody testing for additional autoimmunity, including celiac disease (anti-tissue transglutaminase 2 antibodies, antigliadin antibodies, both immunoglobulin G [IgG] and IgA) and autoimmune thyroiditis (anti-thyroperoxidase antibodies, anti-thyroid-stimulating hormone receptor antibodies), was consistently negative. Since neonatal diabetes mellitus is a rare condition that almost invariably recognizes a monogenic cause, with recessive forms more frequently found in consanguineous families [1, 2], direct DNA sequencing of the most common permanent neonatal diabetes mellitus genes (i.e., KCNJ11, INS, and ABCC8) was performed by the standard Sanger method, revealing a homozygous c.3G > A (p.Met1Ile; INSATG>ATA) mutation. The mutation found in our patient is predicted to abrogate insulin translation initiation and cause a permanent form of NDM [12]. At the time of the study, the patient was 11 years old. He was reported to be overweight (height: 126.8 cm; weight: 41.5 kg; BMI: 25.8) and free from any diabetic-related complications. His treatment regimen consisted of insulin therapy at a medium dose (0.66 UI/kg/day). His HbA1c level from age 3–11 years was reported to range between 7.1% and 9.1% (54–76 mmol/mol).

Obtaining a skin biopsy from our patient, after parental informed consent and derived fibroblast cultures, in the study of Ma et al. [13], were generated induced pluripotent stem cells.

Differentiation of mutant cells resulted in insulin-negative endocrine stem cells expressing MAFA, NKX6.1, and chromogranin A. Correction of the mutation in stem cells and differentiation to pancreatic endocrine cells restored insulin production and insulin secretion to levels comparable to those of wild-type cells. Grafting of corrected cells into mice, followed by ablating mouse b cells using streptozotocin, resulted in normal glucose homeostasis, including at night, and the stem cell-derived grafts adapted insulin secretion to metabolic changes.

The study made on patient's fibroblasts lays the foundation for the generation of genetically corrected cells autologous from a patient with non-autoimmune insulin-dependent diabetes.

Cases that might be readily amenable to autologous cell therapy [13].

5.1.4 Case #4

This is the case of a child born in September 2012.

During the pregnancy (30th week) the gynecologist noted polyhydramnios and a doubled gastric bubble, with growth around the 5th centile.

He was born with vaginal delivery at 38 + 3 weeks of gestational age from the first pregnancy, without complication except for a vaginal swab positive for *S. agalactiae* (treated with Ampicillin-Sulbactam before delivery). No familiar history of diabetes or other diseases. Apgar was 9 at first and 9 in the fifth minute. At first visit, weight was 2.040 kg (<3° centile, −2.7 SDS), length 44.6 cm (<3° centile, −2.36 SDS), cranial circumference was 31.2 cm (<3° centile, −2.34 SDS). The general appearance was good, with HR 150 bpm, normal peripheral pulses, no abdominal masses, normal breathing, pulse oximetry 100%, with no abnormalities in palate, pharynx, and anus. Normal tone and reflex were evident. A mild metabolic acidosis was evident (pH 7.167, pCO_2 56.9 mmHg, HOC_3–19.8 mmol/L, BE −7.5 mmol/L), and 2 ml of bicarbonates were given intravenously. A nasogastric tube was placed, and glucose was commenced through the intravenous route (4 ml/h).

On the first day of life, the abdomen radiograph evaluation confirmed the diagnosis of duodenal stenosis/atresia. On the second day of life, the child underwent surgical intervention of duodenum-duodenal anastomosis and appendicectomy, with the correction of duodenal atresia. Partial intestinal malrotation (cecal intestine was free in mesogastrium) was also noted. The post-intervention course was regular, except for variable hyperglycemia (110–299 mg/dl (6.11–16.59 mmol/L)) while he had been receiving parenteral nutrition, with a recommendation of moderate glucose restriction in the nutritional bag.

Three weeks after the surgical intervention, progressive emesis (also biliary) appeared, therefore a transit study and an esophagogastroduodenoscopy revealed a block in the jejune; therefore, he received a surgical revision, with adherences lysis, jejunal resection and termino-terminal jejune-jejunal anastomosis, and he began to be fed with donated breastfeed milk after 3 weeks, without other complications. Hyperglycemia reduced, and values between 110 and 140 mg/dl (6.11–7.77 mmol/L) were noted in the following weeks, with a diagnosis of stress-related hyperglycemia. He received some blood (red blood cells and platelets) transfusion for anemia and low platelet count.

He was discharged at 4 months of life in good condition, with normal cardiac and abdominal ultrasound, normal thyroid function, normal blood cells count, and mild neurologic retardation, with a weight of 3.450 kg.

At 5 months of age, he was readmitted to our Hospital for the appearance of vomit and diarrhea and was discharged 1 month later with a diagnosis of gastroenteritis. During the admission, moderate hyperglycemia was noted, thus home glucose monitoring was recommended.

At 9 months of age, the mother observed some glycemic values above 300 mg/dL (16.65 mmol/L). The child was then admitted and at laboratory evaluation, we encountered a value of C-peptide below the normal range (0.99 ng/mL, normal value 1.10–4.40) and an HbA1c value of 8%. In the suspect of monogenic diabetes, we decided to commence insulin therapy with an insulin pump together with continuous glucose monitoring (CGM, Dexcom G4, San Diego, USA), but we had to stop insulin since glycemic values returned to normal. We decided to continue CGM at home, and since the appearance of hyperglycemia after meals and during the night, 3 weeks after we restarted insulin at a low dose (0.15 UI/kg/day), reduced thereafter and maintained only at meals.

In the following years, the child showed multiple episodes of vomit and blood in stool, some of them complicated with anemia treated with blood transfusion, with normal instrumental (radiologic, ultrasound, endoscopic) evaluations. In the suspect of a syndrome, we performed genetic testing including monogenic diabetes, intestinal malformation, and bleeding, with evidence of punctual mutation in exon 10 in RFX6 gene, suspect for Mitchell-Riley syndrome [14, 15]. We investigated duodenal mucosa, and heterotopic gastric epithelium with regenerative hyperplasia was found at histological examination. Similar observation has been made in small intestine, and the child is now evaluated regularly in order to find and remove area of brittle mucosa with gastric metaplasia, to avoid further episodes of anemization.

5.1.5 Case #5

Mutations in the PDX1 gene are a rare cause of NDM associated with pancreatic agenesis [16–23]. We present a case of permanent neonatal diabetes mellitus with exocrine pancreas manifestations and cholestasis due to compound heterozygosity on PDX1 gene.

Our patient was born by cesarean section in a peripheral Hospital and transferred during her 23rd day of life at our University Hospital. She was assisted in the neonatal intensive care unit during her first 4 months of life.

She was a Caucasian girl and the second child of not consanguineous parents.

Her mother did not have a history of gestational diabetes but she reported taking metformin in the past and she is currently being treated for high blood pressure and hypothyroidism. No one else had diabetes mellitus in their family.

Our patient was born at 34 weeks of gestation with a birth weight of 1180 g (<third percentile) and a length of 40 cm (<third percentile).

The clinical examinations revealed heart rate (HR) of 90 beats per minute and desaturation of Peripheral Oxygen (spO_2) with respiratory distress syndrome (RDS) and continuous positive airway pressure (CPAP) was used to assist the newborn.

On the second day of life, she presented sloping edema and hypocholic stools.

An ultrasound of our patient revealed a small and dysmorphic gallbladder, normal liver, spleen, and pancreas not evaluable. Echocardiography showed a patent foramen ovale (PFO). Ultrasound of her brain revealed diffuse hyperechogenicity of the cerebral and cerebellar parenchyma.

Blood examination on the first day (day of birth) showed hyperglycemia (Gly 7.67 mmol/L), anemia (Hb 7.6 gr/dl), and neonatal cholestasis (GGT 1619 IU/L). On the second day of life, the glycemic value was 26.78 mmol/L, hypoalbuminemia (Albumin 2.20 gr/dl) and hypertrasaminasemia (ALT 82 IU/L; AST 517 IU/L) were revealed.

Fecal elastase (7 mcg/g) and Steatocrit (23%) dosages were indicative of severe exocrine pancreas insufficiency.

Nuclear Magnetic Resonance (NMR) imaging of the abdomen showed an enlarged liver, small and dysmorphic gallbladder, and pancreatic parenchyma visible only at the cephalic level.

Genetic analysis detected a compound heterozygosity on PDX1 gene on chromosome 13 (c.452 C > T and c.587A > C) (p.[THr151Met];[Asn196Thr]).

The missense variant p.[THr151Met] with paternal segregation has an allelic frequency equal to 0.000007131 in the general population (gnomAD) it is not reported in the scientific literature and can be classified as a variant of uncertain significance (ACMG: VUS Class 3). The missense variant p.[Asn196Thr]) with maternal segregation has an allelic frequency equal to 0.00002790 in the general population (gnomAD) it is not reported in the scientific literature and can be classified as a variant of uncertain significance (ACMG: VUS Class 3). These variants were confirmed by Sanger sequencing.

Pathogenetic variants of the PDX1 gene are associated with neonatal diabetes and pancreatic developmental abnormalities with autosomal recessively inherited (OMIM: 260370).

On the second day, neonatal diabetes mellitus was diagnosed as having hyperglycemia (serum glucose level was 7.6 mmol/L) by blood examination and treatment with insulin infusion rates were regularly titrated according to pre-prandial blood sugar levels (0.2 UI/kg/h almost 4 unit/kg per day) and parenteral nutrition with glucose intake of 4 mg/kg/min; the type of lactation was fortified formula. On the third day, due to poor glycemic control, it was started regular daily insulin injections (1 unit/kg per day) with human regular insulin administered every 4 h subcutaneously.

Other treatment operations included infant oxygen hood (oxyhood), nasal continuous positive airway pressure (nCPAP), broad-spectrum antibiotics prescription, red blood cell (RBC) transfusions, ursodeoxycholic acid (UDCA), fat-soluble vitamins prescription, and total parenteral nutrition (TPN) for 23 days.

On the 23rd day of life, at the University Hospital, a sensor-augmented pump (SAP) therapy, MiniMed 640G insulin pump with SmartGuard® (Low Glucose Suspend algorithm), was started.

At this link, we show the moment of implantation of the pump

https://www.dropbox.com/s/wk9a3e183fjio5z/VIDEO-2021-04-26-16-39-10.mp4?dl=0

The insulin dosage was kept low in the first days of the new therapy (0.2 U/kg per day) to reach stable levels throughout the observation period (1 U/kg per day). The sensor glucose average was stable for 30 days of observation (10.56 mmol/L) and the Time in Range (3.89–10 mmol/L) was 58%. Time below Range (<3.89 mmol/L) was 4%.

The association between neonatal diabetes and anemia (Thiamine Responsive Megaloblastic Anemia syndrome) led to therapy with Thiamine (27 mg twice daily), pending the response of genetic investigations, in an attempt to cause the remission of anemia and at the same time also of diabetes mellitus. No subsequent transfusions were required but no effect was seen on glycemic control.

Therapy for pancreatic exocrine insufficiency was oral pancreatic enzymes.

Due to the persistence of cholestasis indices (hyperbilirubinemia, hypertransaminasemia, hyper GGT) in the suspicion of biliary tract atresia, the patient was transferred to pediatric surgery where this diagnosis was excluded, especially due to the sudden improvement in cholestasis indices.

The genetic diagnosis was then completed (PDX1 gene mutation). It was suspended thiamine therapy and it was confirmed insulin pump therapy (permanent neonatal diabetes mellitus), oral pancreatic enzymes, fat-soluble vitamins prescription (pancreatic exocrine insufficiency), and ursodeoxycholic acid (cholestasis).

Currently, the patient (9 months old) has excellent weight growth, good neurological performance, and excellent glycemic control (Fig. 5.1). Sensor-augmented insulin pumps (SAP) therapy has proven to be safe and effective in treating diabetes in this patient and certainly represents the central point of the therapeutic success obtained.

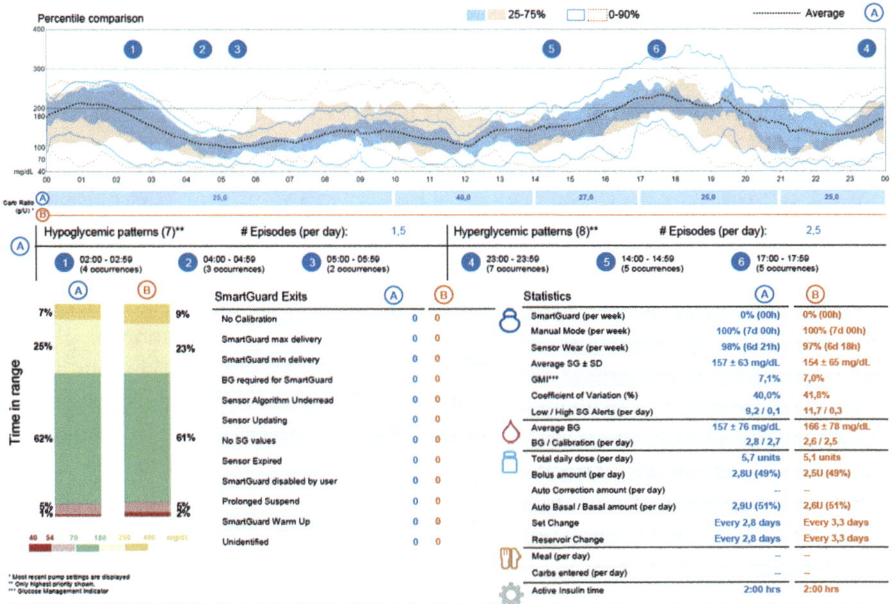

Fig. 5.1 Current glycemic control (9 months of life) in a patient with permanent neonatal diabetes due to a mutation of the PDX1 gene on therapy with MiniMed insulin pump with SmartGuard®

5.1.6 *Case #6*

RD, female, a term-born baby, small for gestational age (2510 g), at age of 2 months was admitted to our Center of Pediatric Diabetes for diabetic ketoacidosis (DK). Laboratory investigations showed: glycemia 38.02 mmol/l, blood ketones 7 mmol/l, PH 7.05; HCO_3–6 mmol/l; BE −23 mmol/l; and hemoglobin glycosylated 6.3%, 45 mmol/mol. Autoantibodies related to autoimmune diabetes [antibodies to Glutamic Acid Decarboxylase 65 (GAD-65), to Zinc Carrier 8 (ZnT8), to pancreatic insula (ICA) and insulin (IAA)] were negative. She was treated with intravenous rehydration and insulin therapy according to Italian Society of Pediatric Endocrinology and Diabetology (ISPED) recommendations of DK treatment [24]. A clinical diagnosis of NDM was made. After resolution of DK, insulin therapy was administered via subcutaneous insulin infusion at a dose of 1.5–2 UI/kg/day.

Due to the high risk of hyperglycemia and hypoglycemia, a continuous glucose monitoring system (CGMS) with low glucose predictive alarms (Dexcom G6 sensor) was started [25–28].

The genetic testing showed a c.620G > A, p.R201H mutation of KCNJ11 (KIR 6.2) gene and SU therapy was started. At the age of 3 months, to obtain the switch from insulin to SU, glibenclamide therapy was started at a dose of 0.16 mg/kg/day into four administrations and gradually increased up to 0.32 mg/kg/day, while insulin was gradually reduced until to suspension.

In order to evaluate glycemic control and glucose variability glucometrics were analyzed [29].

The CGM data showed: mean sensor glucose (SG) 108 mg/dL, SD 28 mg/dL, CV 26%, and GMI 5.4%, percent SG at <54 mg/dL 1.1%, <70 mg/dL 5.2%, time in range (TIR) (≥70–180 mg/dL) 92.6%, time above range (TAR) >180 mg/dL 1%, and TAR >250 mg/dL 0.1%.

Since the Glibenclamide was only available in tablet form, a 5-mg/ml of galenic suspension was prepared, with the indication to keep the solution in the refrigerator at 4 °C and shaking the solution before use.

After 1 week, hypoglycemia occurred (38 mg/dl) and the dose of glibenclamide was reduced at 0.2 mg/kg/day administered thanks to further dilution of glibenclamide to 1.25 mg/ml. The glucometrics of the child was analyzed by our center every week, through telemedicine consultations. By the age of 5 months, the patient had grown adequately and had normal psychomotor development. Subsequently, because of recurring hypoglycemia episodes, SU was reduced firstly to 0.03 mg/kg/day, and 30 days after to 0.027 mg/kg/day on the basis of the glucometrics analysis. During the follow-up, the child required additional and progressively lower dosages of SU, and continued changes in drug dilution (0.625 mg/ml; 0.3 mg/ml). At present, the child is 21 months old, weight 12 kg, SU dose is 0.0037 mg/kg/day in 3 administrations/day. The CGM data show: SG 124 mg/dL, SD 30 mg/dL, CV 24%, and GMI 6.3%, percent SG at <54 mg/dL 0.3%, <70 mg/dL 1%, time in range (TIR) (≥70–180 mg/dL) 94%, time above range (TAR) >180 mg/dL 4.5%, and TAR >250 mg/dL 0.2%, Dilution of SU is 0.3 mg/ml. The baby is in well-being, with normal growth and with normal psychomotor development by age.

The SU dosage required by our case affected by NDM due to a KCNJ11 mutation appears to be the lowest described by literature (Table 5.1). Indeed, the cases described report a dose of 0.1–1.45 mg/kg/day (median 0.4), except for one child who required 0.017 mg/kg/day at the age of 9 months [30]. In this latter case, the authors suggested that the low required dose could be due to the early start of SU treatment at the age of 5 days. Surprisingly, the child was affected by the same c.620G > A, p.R201H mutation of the KCNJ11 gene.

As suggested by Letourneau et al. [31], the successful switch from insulin therapy to SU could have been due to the young age at which was started SU.

In our case, after the good response to the switch to SU, it was not easy to administer the right dose of SU using the available pharmaceutical form, due to both the instability of the preparation itself and the minimum required dosage of the patient.

It would be desirable to have the availability also in Italy of Glibenclamide in the form of oral suspension, as already available in France, where it was found to be effective and safe in patients with NDM [32].

Based on our experience, we agree with various results of literature highlighting the usefulness of CGM in infants with NDM [25, 28, 29]. The CGM allows to control the glycemic instability and it determines an optimal titration of the required dose of the drug. In addition, CGM sensors remove the discomfort of the capillary control, possessing a high sensitivity (94.6%) and specificity (97.9%) even in

Table 5.1 SU doses in NDM due to KCNJ11 mutation in the literature

References	Patients (*n*)	SU dose mg/kg/day
Ahn 2015 [34]	1	0.3
Al-Mahdi 2010 [35]	1	0.1–0.8
Babiker 2016 [36]	127	>0.8
Battaglia 2012 [37]	1	0.09–0.37
Beltrand 2019 [32]	10[a]	0.13
Bowman 2018 [26]	81	0.1–0.6
Chai-Udom 2016 [38]	1	0.85
Cho 2017 [39]	1	2.4
Doneray 2014 [40]	1	0.6
Dupont 2012 [41]	1	0.1–0.8
Ganesh 2016 [42]	1	0.5
Globa 2015 [43]	7	0.075–1.1
Heo 2013 [44]	1	0.1–2.2
Hicks 2014 [45]	2	0.06–0.7
Iocara 2017 [46]	1	0.6–2.6
Itoh 2013 [47]	1	0.2–2
Jahnavi 2013 [48]	4	0.3–0.5
Jain 2017 [49]	3	0.9–2
Ješić 2011 [50]	1	0.12-0.3
Joshi 2011 [51]	1	0.1–0.4
Lanning 2018 [52]	30	Median 0.39
Lau 2015 [53]	1	1.6
Li 2017 [54]	10	0.3–0.8
Madani 2016 [55]	1	0.5–0.8
Mohamadi 2010 [56]	1	0.1–1.45
Nyangabyaki-Twesigye 2015 [57]	1	0.9–1.6
Peña-Almazan 2015 [58]	1	1.2–1.9
Philla 2013 [59]	1	0.4
Russo 2011 [60]	1	0.28
Wambach 2010 [30]	1	0.017
Yang 2013 [61]	1	0.1–1
Yoon 2018 [62]	1	0.6
Zhang 2015 [63]	5	0.18–0.54

[a] Not specified if ABCC8 or KCNJ11 patients

premature patients compared to the capillary [28] avoiding performing an elevated number of self-monitoring of blood glucose [33].

Modern CGM sensors have predictive alarms for hypoglycemia, that represent a protective way to follow this particular kind of children affected by NDM, which usually appear asymptomatic in case of hypoglycemia in the first months of life.

References

1. Polak M, Cave H. Neonatal diabetes mellitus: a disease linked to multiple mechanisms. Orphane J RareDis. 2007;2(1):12–23.
2. Barbetti F, Mammì C, Liu M, et al. Neonatal diabetes: permanent neonatal diabetes and transient neonatal diabetes. In: Diabetes associated with single gene defects and chromosomal abnormalities. Vol 25. S. Karger AG; 2017:1–25. https://doi.org/10.1159/000454748
3. Verbsky JW, Chatila TA. Immune dysregulation, polyendocrinopathy, enteropathy, X-linked (IPEX) and IPEX-related disorders: an evolving web of heritable autoimmune diseases. Curr Opin Pediatr. 2013;25(6):708–14. https://doi.org/10.1097/MOP.0000000000000029.
4. Myers AK, Perroni L, Costigan C, Reardon W. Clinical and molecular findings in IPEX syndrome. Arch Dis Child. 2006;91(1):63–4. https://doi.org/10.1136/adc.2005.078287.
5. Goudy K, Aydin D, Barzaghi F, et al. Human IL2RA null mutation mediates immunodeficiency with lymphoproliferation and autoimmunity. Clin Immunol. 2013;146(3):248–61. https://doi.org/10.1016/j.clim.2013.01.004.
6. Caudy AA, Reddy ST, Chatila T, Atkinson JP, Verbsky JW. CD25 deficiency causes an immune dysregulation, polyendocrinopathy, enteropathy, X-linked-like syndrome, and defective IL-10 expression from CD4 lymphocytes. J Allergy Clin Immunol. 2007;119(2):482–7. https://doi.org/10.1016/j.jaci.2006.10.007.
7. Barzaghi F, Passerini L, Gambineri E, et al. Demethylation analysis of the FOXP3 locus shows quantitative defects of regulatory T cells in IPEX-like syndrome. J Autoimmun. 2012;38(1):49–58. https://doi.org/10.1016/j.jaut.2011.12.009.
8. Yong PL, Russo P, Sullivan KE. Use of sirolimus in IPEX and IPEX-like children. J Clin Immunol. 2008;28(5):581–7. https://doi.org/10.1007/s10875-008-9196-1.
9. Romano F, Tinti D, Spada M, Barzaghi F, Rabbone I. Neonatal diabetes in a patient with IPEX syndrome: an attempt at balancing insulin therapy. Acta Diabetol. 2017;54(12):1139–41.
10. Halabi-Tawil M, Ruemmele FM, Fraitag S, et al. Cutaneous manifestations of immune dysregulation, polyendocrinopathy, enteropathy, X-linked (IPEX) syndrome. Br J Dermatol. 2009;160(3):645–65.
11. Passerini L, Barzaghi F, Curto R, Sartirana C, Barera G, Tucci F, et al. Treatment with rapamycin can restore regulatory T-cell function in IPEX patients. Allergy Clin Immunol. 2020;145(4):1262–1271.e13. https://doi.org/10.1016/j.jaci.2019.11.043.
12. Garin I, Edghill EL, Akerman I, et al. Recessive mutations in the INS gene result in neonatal diabetes through reduced insulin biosynthesis. Proc Natl Acad Sci U S A. 2010;107(7):3105–10. https://doi.org/10.1073/pnas.0910533107.
13. Ma S, Viola R, Sui L, Cherubini V, Barbetti F, Egli D. β cell replacement after gene editing of a neonatal diabetes-causing mutation at the insulin locus. Stem Cell Rep. 2018;11(6):1407–15. https://doi.org/10.1016/j.stemcr.2018.11.006.
14. Zegre Amorim M, Houghton JA, Carmo S, Salva I, Pita A, Pereira-da-Silva L. Mitchell-Riley syndrome: a novel mutation in RFX6. Gene Case Rep Genet. 2015;2015:9372.
15. Kambal MA, Al-Harbi DA, Al-Sunaid AR, Al-Atawi MS Mitchell-Riley syndrome due to a novel mutation in RFX6. Front Pediatr. 2019;7:243. https://doi.org/10.3389/fped.2019.00243. eCollection 2019.
16. De Franco E, Shaw-Smith C, Flanagan SE, Edghill EL, Wolf J, Otte V, et al. Biallelic PDX1 (insulin promoter factor 1) mutations causing neonatal diabetes without exocrine pancreatic insufficiency. Diabet Med. 2013;30:e197–20.
17. Sahebi L, Niknafs N, Dalili H, Amini E, Esmaeilnia T, Amoli M, Farrokhzad N. Iranian neonatal diabetes mellitus due to mutation in PDX1 gene: a case report. J Med Case Rep. 2019;13(1):258.
18. Nicolino M, Claiborn KC, Senée V, Boland A, Stoffers DA, Julier C. A novel hypomorphic PDX1 mutation responsible for permanent neonatal diabetes with subclinical exocrine deficiency. Diabetes. 2010;59(3):733–40.

19. Kulkarni A, Sharma VK, Nabi F. PDX1 gene mutation with permanent neonatal diabetes mellitus with annular pancreas, duodenal atresia, hypoplastic gall bladder and exocrine pancreatic insufficiency. Indian Pediatr. 2017;54(12):1052–3.
20. De Franco E, Shaw-Smith C, Flanagan SE, Edghill EL, Wolf J, Otte V, Ebinger F, Varthakavi P, Vasanthi T, Edvardsson S, Hattersley AT, Ellard S. Biallelic PDX1 (insulin promoter factor 1) mutations causing neonatal diabetes without exocrine pancreatic insufficiency. Diabet Med. 2013;30(5):e197–200.
21. Chen R, Hussain K, Al-Ali M, Dattani MT, Hindmarsh P, Jones PM, Marsh P. Neonatal and late-onset diabetes mellitus caused by failure of pancreatic development: report of 4 more cases and a review of the literature. Pediatrics. 2008;121(6):e1541–7.
22. Ashraf A, Abdullatif H, Hardin W, Moates JM. Unusual case of neonatal diabetes mellitus due to congenital pancreas agenesis. Pediatr Diabetes. 2005 Dec;6(4):239–43.
23. Melloul D, Tsur A, Zangen D. Pancreatic duodenal Homeobox (PDX-1) in health and disease. J Pediatr Endocrinol Metab. 2002;15(9):1461–72.
24. Raccomandazioni per la gestione della chetoacidosi diabetica in età pediatrica. Acta Biomed. 2015;86(1). ISSN: 0392-4203.
25. Dahl A, Kumar S. Recent advances in neonatal diabetes. Diabetes Metab Syndr Obes. 2020;13:355–64. https://doi.org/10.2147/DMSO.S198932.
26. Bowman P, Sulen Å, Barbetti F, Beltrand J, Svalastoga P, Codner E, et al. Neonatal Diabetes International Collaborative Group. Effectiveness and safety of long-term treatment with sulfonylureas in patients with neonatal diabetes due to KCNJ11 mutations: an international cohort study. Lancet Diabetes Endocrinol. 2018;6(8):637–46. https://doi.org/10.1016/S2213-8587(18)30106-2
27. Stanik J, Dankovcikova A, Barak L, Skopkova M, Palko M, Divinec J, Klimes I, Gasperikova D. Sulfonylurea vs insulin therapy in individuals with sulfonylurea-sensitive permanent neonatal diabetes mellitus, attributable to a KCNJ11 mutation, and poor glycaemic control. Diabet Med. 2018;35(3):386–91. https://doi.org/10.1111/dme.13575.
28. McKinlay CJD, Chase JG, Dickson J, Harris DL, Alsweiler JM, Harding JE. Continuous glucose monitoring in neonates: a review. Matern Health Neonatol Perinatol. 2017;3:18. https://doi.org/10.1186/s40748-017-0055-z.
29. Piona C, Marigliano M, Mozzillo E, Franzese A, Zanfardino A, Iafusco D, Maltoni G, Zucchini S, Delvecchio M, Maffeis C. Long-term glycemic control and glucose variability assessed with continuous glucose monitoring in a pediatric population with type 1 diabetes: determination of optimal sampling duration. Pediatr Diabetes. 2020;21(8):1485–92. https://doi.org/10.1111/pedi.13115.
30. Wambach JA, Marshall BA, Koster JC, White NH, Nichols CG. Successful sulfonylurea treatment of an insulin-naïve neonate with diabetes mellitus due to a KCNJ11 mutation. Pediatr Diabetes. 2010;11(4):286–8. https://doi.org/10.1111/j.1399-5448.2009.00557.x.
31. Letourneau LR, Greeley SAW. Precision medicine: long-term treatment with sulfonylureas in patients with neonatal diabetes due to KCNJ11 mutations. Curr Diab Rep. 2019;19(8):52. https://doi.org/10.1007/s11892-019-1175-9.
32. Beltrand J, Baptiste A, Busiah K, et al. Glibenclamide oral suspension: suitable and effective in patients with neonatal diabetes. Pediatr Diabetes. 2019;20(3):246–54. https://doi.org/10.1111/pedi.12823.
33. Scaramuzza A, et al. Diabetes Study Group of the Italian Society for Pediatric Endocrinology and Diabetology. Recommendations for self-monitoring in pediatric diabetes: a consensus statement by the ISPED. Acta Diabetol. 2014;51(2):173–84. https://doi.org/10.1007/s00592-013-0521-7.
34. Ahn SY, Kim GH, Yoo HW. Successful sulfonylurea treatment in a patient with permanent neonatal diabetes mellitus with a novel KCNJ11 mutation. Korean J Pediatr. 2015;58(8):309–12. https://doi.org/10.3345/kjp.2015.58.8.309.
35. Al-Mahdi M, Al Mutair A, Al Balwi M, Hussain K. Successful transfer from insulin to oral sulfonylurea in a 3-year-old girl with a mutation in the KCNJ11 gene [published correction

appears in Ann Saudi Med. 2010 May-Jun;30(3):242]. Ann Saudi Med. 2010;30(2):162–4. https://doi.org/10.4103/0256-4947.60526.
36. Babiker T, Vedovato N, Patel K, et al. Successful transfer to sulfonylureas in KCNJ11 neonatal diabetes is determined by the mutation and duration of diabetes. Diabetologia. 2016;59(6):1162–6. https://doi.org/10.1007/s00125-016-3921-8.
37. Battaglia D, Lin YW, Brogna C, et al. Glyburide ameliorates motor coordination and glucose homeostasis in a child with diabetes associated with the KCNJ11/S225T, del226-232 mutation. Pediatr Diabetes. 2012;13(8):656–60. https://doi.org/10.1111/j.1399-5448.2012.00874.
38. Chai-Udom R, Sahakitrungruang T, Wacharasindhu S, Supornsilchai V. A girl with permanent neonatal diabetes due to KCNJ11 mutation presented with Mauriac syndrome after improper adjustment in sulfonylurea dosage over 6 years. J Pediatr Endocrinol Metab. 2016;29(9):1095–101. https://doi.org/10.1515/jpem-2016-0065.
39. Cho JH, Kang E, Lee BH, Kim GH, Choi JH, Yoo HW. DEND syndrome with heterozygous KCNJ11 mutation successfully treated with sulfonylurea. J Korean Med Sci. 2017;32(6):1042–5. https://doi.org/10.3346/jkms.2017.32.6.1042.
40. Doneray H, Houghton J, Tekgunduz KS, Balkir F, Caner I. Permanent neonatal diabetes mellitus caused by a novel mutation in the KCNJ11 gene. J Pediatr Endocrinol Metab. 2014;27(3–4):367–71. https://doi.org/10.1515/jpem-2013-0068.
41. Dupont J, Pereira C, Medeira A, Duarte R, Ellard S, Sampaio L. Permanent neonatal diabetes mellitus due to KCNJ11 mutation in a Portuguese family: transition from insulin to oral sulfonylureas. J Pediatr Endocrinol Metab. 2012;25(3–4):367–70. https://doi.org/10.1515/jpem-2011-0191.
42. Ganesh R, Suresh N, Vasanthi T, Ravikumar KG. Neonatal diabetes: a case series. Indian Pediatr. 2017;54(1):33–6. https://doi.org/10.1007/s13312-017-0993-6.
43. Globa E, Zelinska N, Mackay DJ, et al. Neonatal diabetes in Ukraine: incidence, genetics, clinical phenotype and treatment. J Pediatr Endocrinol Metab. 2015;28(11–12):1279–86. https://doi.org/10.1515/jpem-2015-0170.
44. Heo JW, Kim SW, Cho EH. Unsuccessful switch from insulin to sulfonylurea therapy in permanent neonatal diabetes mellitus due to an R201H mutation in the KCNJ11 gene: a case report. Diabetes Res Clin Pract. 2013;100(1):e1–2. https://doi.org/10.1016/j.diabres.2013.01.016.
45. Hicks KA, Kushner JA, Heptulla R, Ham JN. Permanent neonatal diabetes mellitus in monozygotic twins achieving low-dose sulfonylurea therapy. J Pediatr Endocrinol Metab. 2014;27(1–2):135–8. https://doi.org/10.1515/jpem-2013-0171.
46. Ioacara S, Flanagan S, Fröhlich-Reiterer E, Goland R, Fica S. First case of neonatal diabetes with KCNJ11 Q52R mutation successfully switched from insulin to sulphonylurea treatment. J Diabetes Investig. 2017;8(5):716–9. https://doi.org/10.1111/jdi.12620.
47. Itoh S, Matsuoka H, Yasuda Y, et al. DEND syndrome due to V59A mutation in KCNJ11 gene: unresponsive to sulfonylureas. J Pediatr Endocrinol Metab. 2013;26(1–2):143–6. https://doi.org/10.1515/jpem-2012-0236.
48. Jahnavi S, Poovazhagi V, Mohan V, et al. Clinical and molecular characterization of neonatal diabetes and monogenic syndromic diabetes in Asian Indian children. Clin Genet. 2013;83(5):439–45. https://doi.org/10.1111/j.1399-0004.2012.01939.x.
49. Jain V, Satapathy A, Yadav J, et al. Clinical and molecular characterization of children with neonatal diabetes mellitus at a tertiary Care Center in Northern India. Indian Pediatr. 2017;54(6):467–71. https://doi.org/10.1007/s13312-017-1049-7.
50. Ješić MM, Ješić MD, Maglajlić S, Sajić S, Necić S. Successful sulfonylurea treatment of a neonate with neonatal diabetes mellitus due to a new KCNJ11 mutation. Diabetes Res Clin Pract. 2011;91(1):e1–3. https://doi.org/10.1016/j.diabres.2010.09.027.
51. Joshi R, Phatarpekar A. Neonatal diabetes mellitus due to L233F mutation in the KCNJ11 gene. World J Pediatr. 2011;7(4):371–2. https://doi.org/10.1007/s12519-011-0254-z.
52. Lanning MS, Carmody D, Szczerbiński Ł, Letourneau LR, Naylor RN, Greeley SAW. Hypoglycemia in sulfonylurea-treated KCNJ11-neonatal diabetes: mild-moderate symptomatic episodes occur infrequently but none involving unconsciousness or seizures. Pediatr Diabetes. 2018;19(3):393–7. https://doi.org/10.1111/pedi.12599.

53. Lau E, Correia C, Freitas P, et al. Permanent neonatal diabetes by a new mutation in KCNJ11: unsuccessful switch to sulfonylurea. Arch Endocrinol Metab. 2015;59(6):559–61. https://doi.org/10.1590/2359-3997000000076.
54. Li X, Xu A, Sheng H, et al. Early transition from insulin to sulfonylureas in neonatal diabetes and follow-up: experience from China. Pediatr Diabetes. 2018;19(2):251–8. https://doi.org/10.1111/pedi.12560.
55. Madani HA, Fawzy N, Afif A, Abdelghaffar S, Gohar N. Study of KCNJ11 gene mutations in association with monogenic diabetes of infancy and response to sulfonylurea treatment in a cohort study in Egypt. Acta Endocrinol (Buchar). 2016;12(2):157–60. https://doi.org/10.4183/aeb.2016.157.
56. Mohamadi A, Clark LM, Lipkin PH, Mahone EM, Wodka EL, Plotnick LP. Medical and developmental impact of transition from subcutaneous insulin to oral glyburide in a 15-yr-old boy with neonatal diabetes mellitus and intermediate DEND syndrome: extending the age of KCNJ11 mutation testing in neonatal DM. Pediatr Diabetes. 2010;11(3):203–7. https://doi.org/10.1111/j.1399-5448.2009.00548.x.
57. Nyangabyaki-Twesigye C, Muhame MR, Bahendeka S. Permanent neonatal diabetes mellitus - a case report of a rare cause of diabetes mellitus in East Africa. Afr Health Sci. 2015;15(4):1339–41. https://doi.org/10.4314/ahs.v15i4.37.
58. Peña-Almazan S. Successful transition to sulfonylurea in neonatal diabetes, developmental delay, and seizures (DEND syndrome) due to R50P KCNJ11 mutation. Diabetes Res Clin Pract. 2015;108(1):e18–20. https://doi.org/10.1016/j.diabres.2014.12.010.
59. Philla KQ, Bauer AJ, Vogt KS, Greeley SA. Successful transition from insulin to sulfonylurea therapy in a patient with monogenic neonatal diabetes owing to a KCNJ11 F333L [corrected] mutation [published correction appears in Diabetes Care. 2014 Feb;37(2):588]. Diabetes Care. 2013;36(12):e201. https://doi.org/10.2337/dc13-1690
60. Russo C, Salina A, Aloi C, Iafusco D, Lorini R, d'Annunzio G. Mother and daughter carrying the same KCNJ11 mutation but with a different response to switching from insulin to sulfonylurea. Diabetes Res Clin Pract. 2011;94(2):e50–2. https://doi.org/10.1016/j.diabres.2011.07.039.
61. Yang W, Wei H, Sang Y. KCNJ11 in-frame 15-bp deletion leading to glibenclamide- responsive neonatal diabetes mellitus in a Chinese child. J Pediatr Endocrinol Metab. 2013;26(5–6):591–4. https://doi.org/10.1515/jpem-2012-0133.
62. Yoon JS, Park KJ, Sohn YB, Lee HS, Hwang JS. Successful switching from insulin to sulfonylurea in a 3-month-old infant with diabetes due to p.G53D mutation in KCNJ11. Ann Pediatr. Endocrinol Metab. 2018;23(3):154–7. https://doi.org/10.6065/apem.2018.23.3.154.
63. Zhang M, Chen X, Shen S, et al. Sulfonylurea in the treatment of neonatal diabetes mellitus children with heterogeneous genetic backgrounds. J Pediatr Endocrinol Metab. 2015;28(7–8):877–84. https://doi.org/10.1515/jpem-2014-042.

Chapter 6
Insulin Therapy

Ivana Rabbone, Silvia Savastio, Sara Zanetta, Maria Alessandra Saltarelli, and Stefano Tumini

Abbreviations

CGM	Continuous glucose monitoring
CSII	Continuous subcutaneous insulin infusion
HbA1c	Glycated hemoglobin
IV	Intravenous
IVH	Intraventricular hemorrhage
KATP channel	ATP-dependent potassium channel
MDI	Multiple daily injections
NDM	Neonatal diabetes mellitus
NPH	Neutral protamine hagedorn
PNDM	Permanent neonatal diabetes mellitus
SAP	Subcutaneous augmented pump
SU	Sulfonylurea

Supplementary Information The online version contains supplementary material available at https://doi.org/10.1007/978-3-031-07008-2_6.

I. Rabbone (✉) · S. Savastio · S. Zanetta
Division of Pediatrics, Department of Health Sciences, University of Piemonte Orientale, Novara, Italy
e-mail: ivana.rabbone@uniupo.it

M. A. Saltarelli
Department of Pediatrics, University "G. D'Annunzio Chieti-Pescara", Chieti, Italy

S. Tumini
Department of Maternal and Child Health, UOSD Regional Center of Pediatric Diabetology, Chieti Hospital, Chieti, Italy

I. Rabbone, D. Iafusco (eds.), *Neonatal and Early Onset Diabetes Mellitus*, https://doi.org/10.1007/978-3-031-07008-2_6

6.1 Introduction

Neonatal Diabetes Mellitus (NDM) is a rare form of diabetes defined by the onset of persistent hyperglycemia within the first 6 months of life. It is often caused by a mutation in a single gene affecting development and/or function of pancreatic β cells which then leads to a decrease in the insulin secretion or function [1].

The ATP-dependent potassium channel (KATP channel) plays a central role in stimulating insulin secretion by the pancreatic β cell in response to glucose. At low blood sugar levels, the KATP channels are open (activated) and their activity maintains a hyperpolarized resting membrane potential (around −70 mV). A rise in blood sugar level causes increased passage of glucose into the β cell. Glucose enters the glycolysis pathway, which increases the intracellular ATP concentration. This causes the closure of KATP channels (inhibition), which leads to the intracellular potassium accumulation activating membrane depolarization. This depolarization triggers the voltage-dependent calcium channels, therefore Ca^{2+} ions entering the β cell, enabling exocytosis of the secretion vesicles and release of insulin into the bloodstream [2].

Patients with NDM present an early onset of diabetes generally associated with an intrauterine growth delay. For this reason, the initial treatment should be aimed at rebalancing carbohydrate metabolism and should be started immediately after diagnosis. The treatment consists in the balance between calory and carbohydrate intake to restore normal weight without being excessive (15–18 g/kg/daily carbohydrate). It is important to avoid the risk of future insulin resistance and achieve the correct metabolic equilibrium with a sufficient insulin-based treatment [3, 4]. Insulin-based therapy is difficult to manage due to the very low weight of these neonates; moreover, the therapeutic margins between hypoglycemia and hyperglycemia are small, and both are harmful to the neurological development of the newborn [5].

NDM treatment usually involves initial intravenous (IV) insulin infusion; however, the long-term maintenance of intravenous lines can be problematic in small babies, and this delivery method requires continuous hospitalization [6, 7].

Insulin therapy in infants is challenging, for several reasons. Small insulin doses are required, pens and syringes may be lacking in precision and therefore insulin dilution may be necessary with some risks [8]. Considering the infant small body surface area and the limited administration sites, defects in the insulin absorption rate may be due to the real difficulty to perform effective injections [9].

Moreover, breastfeeding can be very variable, both in duration and in meal volume so it could be difficult to carry out a carbohydrate count with the risk of hypoglycemic episodes. Finally, insulin dose requirements may vary between day and night and over time within patients and some newborns could show an increased insulin sensitivity [8].

Considering these limitations, starting CSII therapy can be advantageous in terms of delivering small doses of insulin with greater precision, avoiding painful injections, and allowing better glucometabolic control [10, 11]. Furthermore, some newer pumps do not require insulin dilution, delivery can be adapted to feeding patterns, parents can be taught to manage the pumps at home with the possibility to use them as Subcutaneous Augmented Pumps (SAPs) together with Continuous Glucose Monitoring (CGM), which is highly recommended for children with diabetes [12]. No clinical trials of CSII in NDM have been reported, but there are cases in literature that suggest the safety and efficacy of its use in NDM treatment [13].

6.2 Management of the Acute Phase of Neonatal Diabetes

The initial management of an infant with persistent hyperglycemia is the reduction in glucose infusion rate to physiologic glucose requirements for an optimum growth and nutrition balance (6–12 mg/kg/min). Conditions like sepsis must be treated and it is recommended to decrease/discontinue medications that lead to hyperglycemia (as epinephrine, norepinephrine, dopamine, glucocorticoids) whenever it is medically safe and possible. If the patient presents dehydration, electrolyte imbalance, or ketoacidosis, intravenous fluids and electrolytes should be administered with close monitoring of liquid balance. Following these measures, the initial treatment foresees intravenous insulin infusion, but in literature guidelines for dosing and titrating insulin in neonates are lacking. In some studies, an initial dose of 0.05 U/kg/h is recommended [14]; in others, effective glucose control is achieved with insulin rates ranging as low as 0.02 U/kg/h. Continuous IV infusion of regular insulin is the treatment of choice [15].

During insulin infusion, blood glucose levels need to be monitored every hour; insulin infusion rates should be adjusted in small increments of 0.01 U/kg/h when glucose levels are less than 100 or greater than 200 mg/dL. Finally, when hyperglycemia is persistent and oral feeding have been established, infants should be transitioned to subcutaneous insulin via multiple daily injections (MDI) or CSII, with blood glucose levels at least above 200–250 mg/dL and administering an initial insulin conservative dose in order to decrease the risk of hypoglycemia.

With MDI therapy, a starting dose of 0.1–0.15 U/kg/dose is recommended, using a rapid-acting insulin analog (aspart or lispro); the treatment is characterized by 3–4 insulin administrations per day before feeding, when blood glucose levels are greater than 200–250 mg/dL [16]. Insulin lispro is approved for use in patients of any age, while insulin aspart and glulisine are only approved for use in children over 2 and 6 years, respectively [17–19].

It is necessary that all preprandial blood glucose values must be checked, at least initially. The smallest dose of subcutaneous insulin that can be administered without dilution is 0.5 U. Smaller doses as low as 0.1 U are possible using dilution of the U-100 insulin (100 U of insulin per 1 mL) to up to one-tenth of the original concentration. Infants can also receive long-acting insulin such as glargine at a dose of 0.2–0.4 unit/kg/day in 1 or 2 injections per day [10, 20]. Total daily insulin requirements can vary from 0.29 U/kg to 1.4 U/kg/day [4]. Intermediate-acting insulins such as regular and Neutral Protamine Hagedorn (NPH) insulin should be avoided due to the increased risk of hypoglycemia, compared with short and long-acting analogs [9]. In addition, for breastfed infants, carbohydrate counting is challenging [21].

As mentioned previously, transition from MDI to CSII therapy in NDM is recommended to reach a better glycemic control and solve insulin delivery problems related to MDI. All pediatric patients with diabetes (including NDM), are candidates for CSII, regardless of age [22]. Short-acting insulin or rapid-acting analogues (e.g., lispro and aspart) are the most used in CSII; rapid-acting insulin analogues are generally considered as the first choice in pumps because they provide a greater reduction in glycated hemoglobin (HbA1c) [23, 24]. Moreover, only insulin lispro is approved for use in patients of any age [19, 25].

The total insulin daily dose is usually 0.2–1.4 U/kg/day of which the basal rate accounts for 20–76%. In literature, we can find that pre-meal boluses generally range from 0.05 to 0.2 U/meal or 0.01–0.1 U per 10–15 g of carbohydrate, insulin correction factor is about 0.1 U for every 100 mg above 150 mg/dL of glycemia and a reduced night-time basal rate is suggested.

There are many case reports about utilization of CSII in NDM [5, 7, 13], from which several aspects can be underlined: the starting age of CSII is usually between 18 and 62 days and the reasons for switching from MDI to CSII therapy are frequent hypoglycemias, wide fluctuations in blood glucose levels and difficulty in maintaining intravenous route. The types of insulin pump mainly reported are MiniMed 508 or 507, Disetronic, Animas, and Paradigm. The different outcomes obtained from the switch to CSII are really relevant: good metabolic control, reduction of severe hypoglycemia and significant complications, good weight gain, reduction in glycemic variability, and easier insulin management. Rabbone et al. described four patients with NDM from Italy; three received IV insulin from 6 to 31 days before transition to insulin lispro CSII. The pumps were programmed with basal rates of between 0.025 and 0.1 U/h, plus meal boluses. Two of the babies presented mutations of the KCNJ11 (Kir 6.2) suggesting PNDM and they were both switched from CSII to glibenclamide; the third infant had a mutation of the INS gene and continued CSII therapy; the fourth patient started insulin lispro CSII at the age of 18 days because blood glucose levels were consistently above 8.9 mmol/L (160 mg/dL). CGM was integrated into three patients. All infants obtained improved glycometabolic control [13].

CSII can be used integrated with CGM as SAP, which is highly recommended for children with type 1 diabetes. Even if data are limited, CGM has proven feasible in babies with NDM, both in the hospital setting and after discharge permitting a frequent control of glucose levels, which is important for optimizing insulin treatment [4, 12]. Moreover, CGM reduces hypoglycemia risk and when integrated with an insulin pump leads to a more precise blood glucose level control in the neonatal period [11]. This is considered a very helpful tool for glucose testing and parental reassurance [26].

6.3 Strategies for Long-Term Management and Transferring to Oral Therapy

Patients with NDM often receive their initial treatment in a neonatal department. The treatment consists of sufficient insulin treatment and a balanced diet in calorie and carbohydrate intake necessary to restore normal weight.

After the acute phase, subjects with ABCC8 or KCNJ11 mutations are treated successfully using hypoglycemic SU. These drugs close the KATP channel in an ATP-independent way binding SUR1 subunit of the potassium channel and restoring insulin secretion in response to a meal [5, 27]. The mutated channels are sensitive to sulfonylureas in 90–95% of cases and insulin therapy generally can be stopped [28].

Glibenclamide is the most used SU drug in patients with NDM. SU therapy could be associated to a risk of hypoglycemia, especially if the infant or child has a reduction of food intake. However, the hypoglycemia risk with SU is reduced in comparison to insulin therapy [29].

Younger age at the start of SU therapy and shorter duration of diabetes are associated with higher success in switching from insulin therapy to SU [30].

Sulfonylurea therapy appears to be safe and could be started before genetic testing results are available. The literature has demonstrated that treatment with SU provides better metabolic control than insulin both normalizing HbA1c and reducing the incidence of hypoglycemia in NDM with ABCC8 or KCNJ11 mutations. Bowman et al. in a 10-year multicenter study of a cohort of patients with KCNJ11 PNDM have shown excellent glycemic control with SU therapy (HbA1c 8.1% before transfer to sulfonylureas and 6.4% at the last follow-up). Only mild transient side effects (diarrhea, nausea, weight loss, reduced appetite, and abdominal pain) were found without reports of severe hypoglycemia [31]. Similar results in other studies on diabetes due to KIR6.2 mutations and sulfonylurea therapy after successfully discontinuing insulin [32].

Moreover, the treatment appears able to improve neurological, neuropsychological, and motor impairment [33, 34]. In particular, the best results occur in cases of early start of therapy because SU drugs cross the blood–brain barrier and link SU receptors expressed in the brain closing the neuronal KATP channels and improving neurological outcomes.

It is important to know that up to 10% of patients with KCNJ11 mutations will not respond to SU and will require insulin lifelong [29].

Several approaches have been utilized for transition from insulin (MDI or CSII) to SU. It is important to consider blood glucose before meals and at bedtime during the transition phase. Moreover, CGM can be helpful in monitoring blood glucose values in neonates.

Pearson and colleagues recommend an initial starting dose of glibenclamide of 0.1 mg/kg/dose twice daily before meals and a blood glucose cut-off of 126 mg/dL for titrating the dose. The dose of glibenclamide can be increased by 0.1 mg/kg/dose to at least 1 mg/kg/day achieved in 5–7 days [32].

Other authors suggest a blood cut-off of 200 mg/dl to titrate the glibenclamide dose to reduce hypoglycemia risk [21].

Long-acting and intermediate-acting insulin analogs must be stopped on day 2 of the transition. The long-acting insulin dose has to be decreased the night before starting glibenclamide. In the case of CSII, the basal insulin should be decreased by 50% before giving the first dose of SU. However, reports in literature on CSII and its role during the switch from insulin to glibenclamide are lacking. Furthermore, the dose of the short-acting insulin must be adjusted according to the preprandial blood glucose. In case of blood glucose >200 mg/dL, the usual dose of short-acting insulin prior to the meal should be given. On the contrary, if blood glucose is <200 mg/dL, the preprandial dose should be reduced by at least 50%. Usually, in SU-responsive subjects, insulin can be discontinued in 5–7 days [21].

6.4 Hyperglycemia in Preterm and Low Birth Weight Infants and Insulin Use

There are alternative causes of hyperglycemia in neonates, which can make the diagnosis of NDM difficult. This is especially true in preterm or low birth weight infants, who very frequently experience disorders in glucose homeostasis. In these patients, initially, hypoglycemia is common, due to limited glycogen and fat stores, associated with high-energy demanding conditions, such as respiratory distress, sepsis, hypoxia, and the difficulties of maintaining normothermia. Subsequently, they often become hyperglycemic because of glucose infusion, a combination of insulin resistance and relative insulin deficiency and medications like steroids, theophylline, and vasoactive agents [35, 36].

The prevalence of hyperglycemia in very low birth weight infants is very high during the first postnatal week, with about one-third of these patients developing this complication, but it has been demonstrated that the prevalence remains high for the first 28 postnatal days with a peak during the second week of life [37]. Hyperglycemia in the early period of life is associated with an increased risk of complications like intraventricular hemorrhage (IVH), sepsis, necrotizing enterocolitis, retinopathy of prematurity, a longer length of hospitalization and death [38]. Therefore, an early diagnosis and treatment are necessary.

Currently, there are no established cut-offs for hyperglycemia in preterm infants, with threshold ranging from 125 mg/dL (7 mmol/L) to 180 mg/dL (10 mmol/L) [14, 36, 39]. Some authors describe hyperglycemia as mild for blood glucose levels between 144 and 180 mg/dL (8–10 mmol/L) and severe for blood glucose levels >180 mg/dL (>10 mmol/L) [40]. Hyperglycemia should also be considered in case of blood glucose levels ≥155 mg/dL (8.6 mmol/L) on ≥2 measures >1 h apart [41]. This wide variation in threshold glucose concentrations combined with the lack of guidelines for insulin treatment and the risk of hypoglycemia, determine differences in clinical hyperglycemia management in preterm infants between different neonatal units and countries.

When hyperglycemia has been recognized, if there are no underlying causes to treat, the two possible options are lowering the glucose infusion rate and insulin therapy. Usually, neonatologists use both strategies, starting with glucose infusion rate reduction, and, if not sufficient, adding insulin.

The association between higher glucose infusion rates and risk for hyperglycemia is still not clear [12, 37], but supports reducing the glucose infusion rate as a treatment strategy. The Neonatal Insulin Therapy in Europe (NIRTURE) trial found no association between intravenous glucose infusion rates and hyperglycemia in 188 very low birth weight infants [14, 39]. On the other hand, some authors documented that preterm infants who received less fluid, carbohydrate, fat, and energy had a lower incidence of hyperglycemia [40, 41]. However, the glucose infusion rate should remain between 6 mg/kg/min and 12 mg/kg/min, since glucose infusion rate lower than 6 mg/kg/min can cause severe growth restriction, while 12 mg/kg/min represent the maximal glucose oxidative capacity and higher infusion rate determine inefficient conversion to fat [35]. Furthermore, decreased fat and carbohydrate and increased protein seem to cause a lower incidence of neonatal hyperglycemia, without changing hypoglycemia [41]. A higher daily amino acid intake in parental nutrition seems to be responsible for better insulin secretion. A comparison between a standard daily amino acid intake of 2.5 g/kg versus a high amino acid intake of 4 g/kg per day showed better glucose control and fewer episodes of hyperglycemia in the second case, with no side effects [42].

Use of insulin as a prevention strategy is not recommended because of the risk of hypoglycemia and death before 28 days [36]. On the contrary, insulin treatment is frequently necessary for very low birth weight infants since it decreases mortality in extremely preterm infants with hyperglycemia and the reduction of glucose infusion alone can be responsible for growth failure [37, 43]. Insulin therapy permits greater calory intake improving utilization of infused glucose better than suppressing endogenous glucose production. It also decreases glycosuria, which may cause the loss of a significant amount of energy (2.9–5.8 kcal/kg per day) because of osmotic diuresis [44]. Furthermore, insulin is a growth factor in the fetal period [36].

The major risk with insulin use is hypoglycemia, but it has been shown that severe hypoglycemia (blood glucose concentration < 40 mg/dL [<2.2 mmol/L]) is rare [36]. Other important limitations are the need for frequent glucose checks and subsequent frequent adjustments to the glucose infusion rate and insulin dosage, which, however, may find a solution in CGM devices. It has been demonstrated that CGM can be effectively combined with the use of insulin and glucose infusion titration in order to improve glycemic control in very preterm infants, increasing time in euglycemia [30, 45].

As for definition, there is a wide variation in treatment threshold, ranging between 144 mg/dL (8 mmol/L) and 252 mg/dL (14 mmol/L) [46]. It is important to consider that blood glucose levels greater than 360 mg/dL are responsible for significant osmotic changes which may cause dehydration, dyselectrolytemia, and IVH [35].

So, it is usually recommended to start insulin therapy when glucose levels are persistently more than 250 mg/dL [21].

Initially, infants are usually managed on IV insulin infusion, at an initial dosage of 0.05 U per kilogram [21]. It is also possible to start with a bolus and subsequently transition to a continuous infusion of 0.01–0.05 U/kg per hour [36]. Other studies suggest insulin infusion rate of 0.02–0.10 U/kg/h [15].

Insulin therapy in very low birth weight infants requires titrating the insulin infusion considering blood glucose levels are monitored every hour. Insulin is typically administered in a small volume of 0.9% saline delivered through an infusion pump. It is recommended to first flush the intravenous tube with the insulin solution in order to prevent insulin from adhering to the binding sites on the tubing or to administer the insulin with a protein solution of 0.25% salt-poor albumin [15]. Insulin infusion rates should be titrated by small increments of 0.01 U per kilogram per hour, decreasing infusion rate if blood glucose levels are <200 mg/dL (11.1 mmol/L), and increasing infusion rate in case of blood glucose levels >250 mg/dL (13.9 mmol/L) [21]. It is not advisable to aim for normoglycemia, because of the risk of hypoglycemia. However, differences in fluid/glucose intake and β cell function and/or insulin sensitivity make it difficult to predict the response of individual infants to any given insulin dose, so dosing should be guided by clinical judgment.

Subcutaneous insulin injections may be advantageous in order to avoid complications related to central venous catheters. The use of subcutaneous long-acting insulin glargine has been described in very low birth weight infants [20, 47]. Barone et al. started subcutaneous insulin Glargine in a 28-week gestational age, 680-g female, after she experienced severe episodes of hypoglycemia with regular insulin infusion and subcutaneous insulin detemir. A dose of 0.27 U/kg/day every 12 h was administered, using a 1:100 dilution of insulin in 0.9% saline with excellent response and discontinuation of therapy after 5 days [47]. A similar strategy was used by Hwang et al. in a 23-week gestational age, 680-g male who was in dexamethasone therapy. Insulin glargine was injected subcutaneously once/day for 5 days starting from a dose of 0.25 U/kg, diluted with 0.9% saline [20]. These cases seem to support the use of subcutaneous insulin glargine in very low birth weight infants, since its action depends on ambient pH and not on the availability of reservoir mass, which can be difficult to evaluate in preterm babies, because of the lack of subcutaneous fat. So, insulin glargine seems to offer a more stable absorption than regular insulin, although literature concerning subcutaneous therapy is still lacking [20].

A new approach in treatment of hyperglycemia in preterm infants is the use of subcutaneous insulin pumps. To date, literature concerning the use of these technologies in NDM is directed to term infants. Muzzy Williamson et al. describe a case of a 23-week of gestational age, 520-g female infants who was successfully treated with a subcutaneous insulin pump used do administer regular insulin [48]. Pump reservoir was filled with regular insulin diluted with 0.9% saline to a final concentration of 25 U/mL, allowing an administrated dose of 0.00625 U/h (0.008 U/kg/h). The reservoir was prepared and refrigerated for at least 6 h prior to administration to allow the insulin to bind to the tubing and the reservoir and during administration it was kept outside of the incubator to minimize degradation of the insulin by the warmth of the incubator. Glucose levels were monitored hourly. The reservoir and tubing were changed daily, and the application site was rotated every 3 days. Because of occasional episodes of hypoglycemia, insulin therapy was modified in 2 h of administration followed by 2 h without insulin, with the start of each infusion cycle coinciding with the start of enteral feeds. Within 48 h, blood glucose levels stabilized [49].

Finally, closed-loop systems may be a potential method to improve glucose control in extremely preterm infants. In a recent clinical trial 21 low birth weight babies were randomly assigned to CGM alone supported by a paper algorithm or to CGM with an additional intervention period of closed-loop CGM. Both treatment groups received treatment with regular insulin in concentration of 5 U/kg in 50 mL of 0.9% saline. Compared with CGM alone, closed-loop intervention showed an increased time of blood glucose levels in the target range chosen of 72–144 mg/dL (4–8 mmol/L) threefold. So, in the context of high-intensity and high-cost setting of neonatal intensive care, these preliminary data seem to support further development of closed-loop systems, with real-time glucose-responsive insulin and dextrose delivery to support the care of these babies [50].

References

1. Iafusco D, Stazi MA, Cotichini R, Cotellessa M, Martinucci ME, Mazzella M, et al. Early onset diabetes study group of the Italian society of paediatric endocrinology and diabetology. Permanent diabetes mellitus in the first year of life. Diabetologia. 2002;45:798–804.
2. Gloyn AL, Pearson ER, Antcliff JF, Proks P, Bruining GJ, Slingerland AS, et al. Activating mutations in the gene encoding the ATP-sensitive Potassium-Channel subunit Kir6.2 and permanent neonatal diabetes. N Engl J Med. 2004;350:1838–49. https://doi.org/10.1056/NEJMoa032922.
3. Rubio-Cabezas O, Hattersley AT, Njølstad PR, Mlynarski W, Ellard S, White N, et al. The diagnosis and management of monogenic diabetes in children and adolescents. Pediatr Diabetes. 2014;15(Suppl 20):47–64. https://doi.org/10.1111/pedi.12192.
4. Karges B, Meissner T, Icks A, Kapellen T, Holl RW. Management of diabetes mellitus in infants. Nat Rev Endocrinol. 2012;8:201–11. https://doi.org/10.1038/nrendo.2011.204.
5. Beltrand J, Busiah K, Vaivre-Douret L, Fauret AL, Berdugo M, Cavé H, Polak M. Neonatal diabetes mellitus. Front Pediatr. 2020;8:540718. https://doi.org/10.3389/fped.2020.540718.
6. Bharucha T, Brown J, McDonnell C, Gebert R, McDougall P, Cameron F, et al. Neonatal diabetes mellitus: Insulin pump as an alternative management strategy. Paediatr Child Health. 2005 Sep-Oct;41(9-10):522–6.
7. Park JH, Kang JH, Lee KH, Kim NH, Yoo HW, Lee DY, et al. Insulin pump therapy in transient neonatal diabetes mellitus. Ann Pediatr Endocrinol Metab. 2013;18:148–51. https://doi.org/10.6065/apem.2013.18.3.148.
8. Beardsall K, Pesterfield CL, Acerini CL. Neonatal diabetes and insulin pump therapy. Arch Dis Child Fetal Neonatal Ed. 2011;96:F223–4. https://doi.org/10.1136/adc.2010.196709.
9. Danne T, Bangstad HJ, Deeb L, Jarosz-Chobot P, Mungaie L, Saboo B, et al. ISPAD clinical practice consensus guidelines 2014. Insulin treatment in children and adolescents with diabetes. Pediatr Diabetes. 2014;15(Suppl 20):115–34. https://doi.org/10.1111/pedi.12184.
10. Passanisi S, Timpanaro T, Lo Presti D, Mammı C, Caruso-Nicoletti M. Treatment of transient neonatal diabetes mellitus: insulin pump or insulin glargine? Our experience. Diabetes Technol Ther. 2014;16:880–4. https://doi.org/10.1089/dia.2014.0055.

11. Rabbone I, Barbetti F, Gentilella R, Mossetto G, Bonfanti R, Maffeis C, et al. Insulin therapy in neonatal diabetes mellitus: a review of the literature. Diabetes Res Clin Pract. 2017;129:126–35. https://doi.org/10.1016/j.diabres.2017.04.007.
12. Phillip M, Danne T, Shalitin S, Buckingham B, Laffel L, Tamborlane W, et al. Use of continuous glucose monitoring in children and adolescents*. Pediatr Diabetes. 2012;13:215–28. https://doi.org/10.1111/j.1399-5448.2011.00849.x.
13. Rabbone I, Barbetti F, Marigliano M, Bonfanti R, Piccinno E, Ortolani F, et al. Successful treatment of young infants presenting neonatal diabetes mellitus with continuous subcutaneous insulin infusion before genetic diagnosis. Acta Diabetol. 2016;53(4):559–65. https://doi.org/10.1007/s00592-015-0828-7.
14. Beardsall K, Vanhaesebrouck S, Ogilvy-Stuart AL, Vanhole C, Palmer CR, Ong K, et al. Prevalence and determinants of hyperglycemia in very low birth weight infants: cohort analyses of the NIRTURE study. J Pediatr. 2010;157(5):715–U39. https://doi.org/10.1016/j.jpeds.2010.04.032.
15. Bottino M, Cowett RM, Sinclair JC. Interventions for treatment of neonatal hyperglycemia in very low birth weight infants. Cochrane Database Syst Rev. 2009;1:CD007453. https://doi.org/10.1002/14651858.CD007453.pub2.
16. Park JH, Shin SY, Shim YJ, Choi JH, Kim HS. Multiple daily injection of insulin regimen for a 10-month-old infant with type 1 diabetes mellitus and diabetic ketoacidosis. Ann Pediatr Endocrinol Metab. 2016;21(2):96–8. https://doi.org/10.6065/apem.2016.21.2.96.
17. Novo Nordisk Limited. NovoRapid PumpCart 100 U/ml: summary of product characteristics. http://www.ema.europa.eu/docs/en_GB/document_library/EPAR_Product_Information/human/000258/WC500030372.pdf
18. Sanofi. Apidra 100 U/ml, solution for injection in a cartridge: summary of product characteristics. http://www.ema.europa.eu/docs/en_GB/document_library/EPAR_Product_Information/human/000557/WC500025250.pdf
19. Lilly E, Limited C. Humalog 100U/ml, solution for injection in vial, Humalog 100U/ml, solution for injection in cartridge, Humalog KwikPen 100U/ml, solution for injection: summary of product characteristics. Basingstoke, UK: Eli Lilly and Company Ltd; 2014.
20. Hwang MJ, Newman R, Philla K, Flanigan E. Use of insulin glargine in the management of neonatal hyperglycemia in an ELBW infant. Pediatrics. 2018;141(Suppl 5):S399–403. https://doi.org/10.1542/peds.2016-1638.
21. Lemelman MB, Letourneau L, Greeley SAW. Neonatal diabetes mellitus: an update on diagnosis and management. Clin Perinatol. 2018;45(1):41–59. https://doi.org/10.1016/j.clp.2017.10.006.
22. Kapellen TM, Heidtmann B, Lilienthal E, Rami-Merhar B, Engler-Schmidt C, Holl RW. Continuous subcutaneous insulin infusion in neonates and infants below 1 year: analysis of initial bolus and basal rate based on the experiences from the German working Group for Pediatric Pump Treatment. Diabetes Technol Ther. 2015;17:872–9. https://doi.org/10.1089/dia.2015.0030.
23. Phillip M, Battelino T, Rodriguez H, Danne T, Kaufman F. European Society for Paediatric Endocrinology, et al. Use of insulin pump therapy in the pediatric age-group: consensus statement from the European Society for Paediatric Endocrinology, the Lawson Wilkins Pediatric Endocrine Society, and the International Society for Pediatric and Adolescent Diabetes, endorsed by the American Diabetes Association and the European Association for the Study of Diabetes. Diabetes Care. 2007;30:1653–62. https://doi.org/10.2337/dc07-9922.
24. Siebenhofer A, Plank J, Berghold A, Jeitler K, Horvath K, Narath M, et al. Short acting insulin analogues versus regular human insulin in patients with diabetes mellitus. Cochrane Database Syst Rev. 2006;2:CD003287. https://doi.org/10.1002/14651858.CD003287.pub4.
25. Pozzilli P, Battelino T, Danne T, Hovorka R, Jarosz-Chobot P, Renard E. Continuous subcutaneous insulin infusion in diabetes: patient populations, safety, efficacy, and pharmacoeconomics. Diabetes Metab Res Rev. 2016;32:21–39. https://doi.org/10.1002/dmrr.2653.

26. Iglesias Platas I, Thió Lluch M, Pociello Almiñana N, Morillo Palomo A, Iriondo Sanz M, Krauel VX. Continuous glucose monitoring in infants of very low birth weight. Neonatology. 2009;95:217–23. https://doi.org/10.1159/000165980.
27. Beltrand J, Elie C, Busiah K, Fournier E, Boddaert N, Bahi-Buisson N, et al. Sulfonylurea therapy benefits neurological and psychomotor functions in patients with neonatal diabetes owing to potassium channel mutations. Diabetes Care. 2015;38:2033–41. https://doi.org/10.2337/dc15-0837.
28. Hattersley AT, Greeley SAW, Polak M, Rubio-Cabezas O, Njølstad PR, Mlynarski W, Castano L, Carlsson A, Raile K, Chi DV, Ellard S, Craig ME. ISPAD clinical practice consensus guidelines 2018: the diagnosis and management of monogenic diabetes in children and adolescents. Pediatr Diabetes. 2018;19(Suppl 27):47–63. https://doi.org/10.1111/pedi.12772.
29. Dahl A, Kumar S. Recent advances in neonatal diabetes. Diabetes Metab Syndr Obes. 2020;13:355–64. https://doi.org/10.2147/DMSO.S198932.
30. Babiker T, Vedovato N, Patel K, et al. Successful transfer to sulfonylureas in KCNJ11 neonatal diabetes is determined by the mutation and duration of diabetes. Diabetologia. 2016;59(6):1162–6. https://doi.org/10.1007/s00125-016-3921-8.
31. Bowman P, Sulen Å, Barbetti F, Beltrand J, Svalastoga P, Codner E, et al. Effectiveness and safety of long-term treatment with sulfonylureas in patients with neonatal diabetes due to KCNJ11 mutations: an international cohort study. Lancet Diabetes Endocrinol. 2018;6(8):637–46. https://doi.org/10.1016/S2213-8587(18)30106-2.
32. Pearson ER, Flechtner I, Njølstad PR, Malecki MT, Flanagan SE, Larkin B, et al. Switching from insulin to oral sulfonylureas in patients with diabetes due to Kir6.2 mutations. N Engl J Med. 2006;355(5):467–77. https://doi.org/10.1056/NEJMoa061759.
33. Slingerland AS, Nuboer R, Hadders-Algra M, Hattersley AT, Bruining GJ. Improved motor development and good long-term glycaemic control with sulfonylurea treatment in a patient with the syndrome of intermediate developmental delay, early-onset generalised epilepsy and neonatal diabetes associated with the V59Mmutation in the KCNJ11 gene. Diabetologia. 2006;49:2559–63. https://doi.org/10.1007/s00125-006-0407-0.
34. Shah RP, Spruyt K, Kragie BC, Greeley SAW, Msall ME. Visuomotor performance in KCNJ11-related neonatal diabetes is impaired in children with DEND-associated mutations and may be improved by early treatment with sulfonylureas. Diabetes Care. 2012;35:2086–8. https://doi.org/10.2337/dc11-2225.
35. Ogilvy-Stuart AL, Beardsall K. Management of hyperglycaemia in the preterm infant. Arch Dis Child Fetal Neonatal Ed. 2010;95(2):F126–31. https://doi.org/10.1136/adc.2008.154716.
36. Ramel S, Rao R. Hyperglycemia in extremely preterm infants. NeoReviews. 2020;21(2):e89–97. https://doi.org/10.1542/neo.21-2-e89.
37. Zamir I, Tornevi A, Abrahamsson T, et al. Hyperglycemia in extremely preterm infants—insulin treatment, mortality and nutrient intakes. J Pediatr. 2018;200:104–110.e1. https://doi.org/10.1016/j.jpeds.2018.03.049.
38. Tottman AC, Alsweiler JM, Bloomfield FH, et al. Relationship between measures of neonatal Glycemia, neonatal illness, and 2-year outcomes in very preterm infants. J Pediatr. 2017;188:115–21. https://doi.org/10.1016/j.jpeds.2017.05.052.
39. Beardsall K, Vanhaesebrouck S, Ogilvy-Stuart AL, Vanhole C, Palmer CR, van Weissenbruch M, Midgley P, Thompson M, Thio M, Cornette L, Ossuetta I, Iglesias I, Theyskens C, de Jong M, Ahluwalia JS, de Zegher F, Dunger DB. Early insulin therapy in very-low-birth-weight infants. N Engl J Med. 2008;359:1873–84. https://doi.org/10.1056/nejmoa0803725.
40. Galderisi A, Facchinetti A, Steil GM, et al. Continuous glucose monitoring in very preterm infants: a randomized controlled trial. Pediatrics. 2017;140(4):e20171162. https://doi.org/10.1542/peds.2017-1162.
41. Tottman AC, Bloomfield FH, Cormack BE, et al. Relationships between early nutrition and blood glucose concentrations in very preterm infants. J Pediatr Gastroenterol Nutr. 2018;66:960–6. https://doi.org/10.1097/MPG.0000000000001929.

42. Stensvold HJ, Lang AM, Strommen K, et al. Strictly controlled glucose infusion rates are associated with a reduced risk of hyperglycaemia in extremely low birth weight preterm infants. Acta Paediatr. 2018;107(3):442–9. https://doi.org/10.1111/apa.14164.
43. Heald A, Abdel-Latif ME, Kent AL. Insulin infusion for hyperglycaemia in very preterm infants appears safe with no effect on morbidity, mortality and long-term neurodevelopmental outcome. J Matern Neonatal Med. 2012;25(11):2415–8. https://doi.org/10.3109/14767058.2012.699115.
44. Alsweiler JM, Harding JE, Bloomfield FH. Tight glycemic control with insulin in hyperglycemic preterm babies: a randomized controlled trial. Pediatrics. 2012;129:639–47. https://doi.org/10.1542/peds.2011-2470.
45. Thomson L, Elleri D, Bond S, et al. Targeting glucose control in preterm infants: pilot studies of continuous glucose monitoring. Arch Dis Child Fetal Neonatal Ed. 2019;104:F353–9. https://doi.org/10.1136/archdischild-2018-314814.
46. Morgan C. The potential risks and benefits of insulin treatment in hyperglycaemic preterm neonates. Early Hum Dev. 2015;91:655–9. https://doi.org/10.1016/j.earlhumdev.2015.08.011.
47. Barone JV, Tillman EM, Ferry RJ Jr, et al. Treatment of transient neonatal diabetes mellitus with subcutaneous insulin glargine in an extremely low birth weight neonate. J Pediatr Pharmacol Ther. 2011;16:291–7. https://doi.org/10.5863/1551-6776-16.4.291.
48. Muzzy Williamson JD, Thurlow B, Mohamed MW, et al. Neonatal hyperglycemia in a preterm infant managed with a subcutaneous insulin pump. Am J Health Syst Pharm. 2020;77:739–44. https://doi.org/10.1093/ajhp/zxaa056.
49. Beardsall K, Thomson L, Elleri D, et al. Feasibility of automated insulin delivery guided by continuous glucose monitoring in preterm infants. Arch Dis Child Fetal Neonatal Ed. 2020;105:F279–84. https://doi.org/10.1136/archdischild-2019-316871.
50. Burattini I, Bellagamba MP, Spagnoli C, et al. Targeting 2.5 versus 4 g/kg/day of amino acids for extremely low birth weight infants: a randomized clinical trial. J Pediatr. 2013;163(5):1278–1282.e1. https://doi.org/10.1016/j.jpeds.2013.06.075.

Chapter 7
Pump Therapy and Use of Technologies

Raffaella Di Tonno, Valeria Castorani, Tara Raouf, Andrea Rigamonti, Giulio Frontino, Valeria Favalli, Elisa Morotti, Federica Sandullo, Claudia Aracu, Francesco Scialabba, and Riccardo Bonfanti

7.1 Introduction

Recent advancements in technology have greatly affected insulin therapy in patients with diabetes. This is represented mostly by the use of Continuous Subcutaneous Insulin Infusion (CSII), and secondly by the introduction of Continuous Glucose Monitoring (CGM) systems [1].

Furthermore, improved glucose control is observed by the combined use of both devices, more specifically sensor-augmented pump therapy (SAP) and automated insulin delivery (closed-loop) systems which allow the release of insulin to be modulated according to glucose trends. "In literature, there is currently strong evidence regarding their safety, effectiveness, and use in children and young adults. However, there is very limited data regarding the use of these devices in the neonatal period" [1–3]. Moreover, as SAP and CGM are currently used in newborns as "off label" devices and their application is at the physician's discretion. It is therefore also mandatory to obtain informed parental consent. The therapeutic management of Neonatal Diabetes Mellitus (NDM) is more challenging than that of children with type 1 diabetes since newborns present peculiar physical, immunological, and metabolic characteristics [4].

Supplementary Information The online version contains supplementary material available at https://doi.org/10.1007/978-3-031-07008-2_7.

R. Di Tonno · V. Castorani · T. Raouf · A. Rigamonti · G. Frontino · V. Favalli · E. Morotti · F. Sandullo · C. Aracu · F. Scialabba · R. Bonfanti (✉)
Pediatric Diabetes Unit, Ospedale San Raffaele, Diabetes Research Institute, Vita Salute University, Milan, Italy
e-mail: ditonno.raffaella@hsr.it; rigamonti.andrea@hsr.it; frontino.giulio@hsr.it; favalli.valeria@hsr.it; morotti.elisa@hsr.it; Sandullo.Federica@hsr.it; Aracu.Claudia@hsr.it; scialabba.francesco@hsr.it; bonfanti.riccardo@hsr.it

I. Rabbone, D. Iafusco (eds.), *Neonatal and Early Onset Diabetes Mellitus*, https://doi.org/10.1007/978-3-031-07008-2_7

In this chapter, we aim to aid physicians involved in the care of NDM by assessing the indications, potential advantages, and limitations of technology applied to these delicate patients.

7.2 Continuous Glucose Monitoring System in Newborns

7.2.1 CGM Functioning and Sensor Types

Currently available CGM devices detect interstitial glucose concentrations subcutaneously at 1-to-15-min intervals using enzyme-tipped electrodes or fluorescence technology. These devices are minimally invasive, as sensors are applied via needle inserters in the subcutaneous tissue or sample transdermal fluid [5].

There are two subcutaneous biosensor types: microdialysis fibers with either external amperometric probe or amperometric needle electrode.

Microdialysis fibers have been used in neonatal care only in research settings, and there are currently no commercial systems available [6]. On the other hand, subcutaneous needle electrodes such as those commercialized by Medtronic Minimed (Northridge, CA, United States) and DexCom (San Diego, CA, United States) have been used for neonatal clinical practice.

7.2.2 Advantages of CGM Use in Neonatal Care

CGM has provided important insights into neonatal care, and interest in its clinical use is consequently ever increasing. Indeed, newborns are frequently exposed to glucose excursions such as hypoglycemic and hyperglycemic episodes, that have been correlated with poorer neurodevelopment in later life [7, 8].

In particular, CGM use may:

- Reduce the frequency of blood sampling allowing for continuous, sensor-based, monitoring.
- Provide a less invasive method as opposed to repeated capillary or blood glucose measurements, which in turn also lowers the risk of infection.
- May promptly detect hypoglycemia or hyperglycemia events and allow timely treatment of episodes.
- Reduces patient discomfort as CGM has been shown to be well-tolerated in infants including very low birth weight (VLBW) newborns.
- Reduce the frequency of local complications which have been reported such as infection, edema, bleeding, or bruising.
- Represents a safe and feasible device for babies with NDM both as inpatients and outpatients.
- It can be integrated with an insulin pump and allow more accurate blood glucose control and easier patient management for the caregiver [9, 10].

To date, literature regarding the routine use of CGM in NDM is lacking. On the contrary, many authors have also described their experience in newborns with a higher risk of hypoglycemia (such as small for gestational age (SGA), intrauterine growth restriction (IUGR), infants of mothers with diabetes, preterm infants, newborns with metabolic, or endocrinological diseases) and hyperglycemia (newborns treated with glucose-containing intravenous fluids, hypoxic-ischemic encephalopathy or sepsis) [11].

The CHYLD Study, a large prospective cohort study of moderate to late preterm infants born at risk of neonatal hypoglycemia evaluated retrospective CGM data for ≥48 h in 75% of the cohort. The authors showed that despite regular blood glucose testing, many infants reported protracted periods of low interstitial glucose (<2.6 mmol/L [<47 mg/dL]) and that nearly 25% of infants with normal blood glucose concentrations had episodes (≥10 min) of low interstitial glucose concentrations detected only on CGM, some of which were prolonged [7]. Of note, when this cohort was reassessed at 4.5 years of age, children who had experienced low glucose concentrations detected by CGM but not by intermittent blood testing had a fourfold increased risk of altered executive function, whereas the risk in those whom hypoglycemia was identified treated was increased only twofold [12].

Also, fully enterally fed preterm babies may have significant glucose fluctuations, varying from hypoglycemia to hyperglycemia within a day, and for several hours at a time [13]. Thus, CGM may also be useful in this context.

It was also shown that a closed-loop system (automatic and CGM-driven insulin delivery) may improve glucose control in extremely preterm infants. This new approach may represent a milestone, providing greater safety and tighter control while minimizing staff time at bedside and changes in fluid/insulin treatment [14].

CGM use alone may greatly improve neonatal glucose control but many limitations have yet to be overcome, such as the accuracy of the device in newborns, the wide variation in insulin sensitivity between babies, the lacking consensus on optimal glucose thresholds in neonatal intensive care, and concerns about increased workload for the nursing staff [15]. Thus, other studies are necessary to clarify these limits and to standardize CGM use.

In practice, sensors may be inserted in the subcutaneous tissue of a newborn's lateral thigh, with additional covering with an occlusive dressing.

7.2.3 *CMG and NDM*

Although data is limited, CGM has also proven feasible in NDM, both in the hospital setting and after discharge [16]. With appropriate alarm settings, it is also possible to predict glucose trends and prevent hypoglycemia. CGM use has become essential as its association with CSII allows to accurately deliver adequate insulin doses both manually and by exploiting closed-loop automatic insulin delivery algorithms [17, 18]. However, infants need sufficient subcutaneous tissue for incorporation of the sensor, and parents must be trained in its data interpretation if CGM is to be continued at home [19].

7.3 Use of CSII in NDM Management

CSII is a therapeutic alternative to Multiple Daily Injections (MDI) for the management of diabetes mellitus also in newborns. CSII allows a more physiological delivery of minute and precise doses of insulin, including a continuous basal infusion which can be adjusted hourly [20].

7.3.1 CSII Characteristics

In short, CSII is an insulin pump that delivers insulin from the reservoir to the subcutaneous tissue through an infusion set. The infusion cannula is placed in the subcutaneous tissue using a spring-loaded needle insertion device and after the set is connected to the pump reservoir, insulin ultimately flows through the infusion set and cannula to the body. Furthermore, the infusion set tubing and the pump may be unclipped from the cannula support attached to the skin, allowing for temporary disconnection when needed.

In the past, CSII did not have the necessary technical characteristics to be applied in newborns (poor subcutaneous tissue, low insulin needs, low carbohydrate meal content, and often unpredictable meal timing). For this reason, in the past, insulin dilution was often necessary. With current new advancements in pump technology, the need to employ dilution is rare if not exceptional [21].

The choice of insulin pumps to be used depends on several factors [20]:

- *The type of insulin* present in the reservoir of CSII are generally regular insulin or rapid-acting insulin analogs (insulin lispro, aspart, and glulisine) [22, 23]. Currently, rapid-acting insulin analogs are mainly used. However, the use of insulin aspart and insulin glulisine is only approved for children over 2 and 6 years of age, respectively [24, 25]. Insulin lispro [26] is approved for use in patients of any age and in children aged over 2 years and adults it shows similar pharmacodynamic profiles [23, 27, 28].
- *Insulin infusion management*: the use of CSII allows small variations in basal insulin infusion rates and some insulin pumps can infuse at rates as low as 0.025 units/h versus the most common 0.05 units/h. Another important advantage of CSII is the possibility to reduce/suspend basal insulin and also to prevent episodes of hypoglycemia [20]. It may also be critical to consider using a pump that can be programmed to deliver no insulin (0.00 units/h) as it may be necessary at certain times of the day [20].
- *Infusion set types*: cannulas of different lengths are available, whose insertion may be oblique or vertical, and manual or with spring-loaded insertion devices. In a newborn, a longer and oblique cannula is preferred because it allows for better anchoring in the subcutaneous tissue, reducing the risk of accidental detachment of the patch [21]. The limited body surface and subcutaneous tissue of the newborn limits the area of skin available for the placement of CSII and could

affect insulin absorption, including the Plissè Effect [29–32]. The choice of infusion site is challenging, especially in low birth weight (LBW) and VLBW newborns, and should be evaluated case by case according to the individual characteristics (gestational age, weight, length, need for additional monitoring). The anterolateral face of the thigh and the superolateral quadrant of the buttock are preferred because they offer more space for insertion, provide more subcutaneous fat, and effective insulin absorption of the infused [21]. Cannulas are often placed near or below the diaper and are therefore exposed to contact with bodily fluids which increases the risk of infusion set detachment and contamination which may be overcome with the use of waterproof adhesive patches [20, 21].

7.3.2 *Insulin Requirements*

When starting CSII therapy daily insulin requirements may often be estimated empirically from:

- The amount of insulin needed in a prior intravenous or MDI treatment phase (with a 20–25% total dose reduction to avoid hypoglycemia) [21].
- The weight of newborn (0.2–0.3 U/Kg/day) [21].

Subsequently, regardless of the type of feeding (breastfed or artificial formula), the daily insulin requirement varies from 0.20 to 1.4 U/Kg/day. Basal insulin in CSII usually accounts for 30% of the daily dose, less than that required in the case of MDI, and boluses account for the remaining 70% [10, 17].

Basal insulin requirements are variable throughout the day, depending on the patient's age. In a child under 1 year of age, the glucose values rise later in the evening and then significantly decrease during the night [4, 33].

Bolus doses (in cases of hyperglycemia or for meals) depend on the insulin-to-carbohydrate ratio (0.01–0.1 Units for every 10–15 grams of carbohydrates or 0.05–0.2 Units per meal) and insulin sensitivity factor (0.1 Units every 100 mg above 150 mg/dL of glycemia [4]. In the case of total parenteral nutrition or continuous enteral feeding, insulin administration mainly through basal infusion is usually required [34].

7.3.3 *Advantages of CSII Use in NDM*

As newborns with NDM require small doses of insulin, the administration is more feasible through the use of CSII rather than MDI. Feeding schedules of infants are often unpredictable and meal duration and quantity are difficult to quantify. These obstacles may be overcome by using the latest generation of pumps which allow a more newborn-tailored insulin administration with fractioned insulin doses and no need for insulin dilution [23, 35, 36].

Recently, many studies have shown that CSII provides better glucose control compared to MDI especially in children and adolescents, as it reduces the risk of both hypoglycemia and diabetic ketoacidosis (DKA) [35, 37–39].

Although data is lacking in newborns, the choice of CSII should naturally be preferred over MDI as supported by data in the study of Fawzia Alyafie et al. showing glycated hemoglobin (HbA1c) improvement in 5 cases of persistent NDM (PDNM) on CSII compared to those on MDI [40].

Furthermore, CSII use is more practical when weaning insulin therapy or when switching from insulin therapy to other treatments, [1, 29] such as in the case of glibenclamide in the case of PDNM in which mutation Kir 6.2 was identified [1].

In conclusion, the advantages of using CSII therapy over MDI therapy can be summarized as follows [23]:

- Fractioned insulin doses.
- No need for insulin dilution.
- Reduced invasiveness: the need for fewer injections in patients with limited body surface area and poorly represented subcutaneous tissue.
- Insulin doses are more tailored to the unpredictable feeding patterns of the newborn.
- Basal insulin may be adjusted hourly to follow variations in daily insulin requirements.
- Improved glucose control.

7.3.4 Pitfalls in CSII Use

The use of the CSII may be associated with an increased risk of DKA due to unrecognized malfunction and/or failure of the device [17]. In the event of pump malfunction due to infusion set/site problems, the latter must be changed and insulin injections may be needed temporarily to avoid progression toward DKA [4].

Another potential complication is infusion site infections [41, 42]. This risk reduces with catheter site changes every 48–72 h and by infusion set insertion in the buttock [17].

The administration of insulin at the same site may cause lipodystrophies, both in the case of insulin MDI therapy and CSII therapy. Insertion site rotation is therefore mandatory [17, 38].

Adequate caregiver education is essential to achieve effective NDM management with CSII and allows to secure all the benefits as well as minimize the potential risks and complications [17].

Consequently, hospitalization for at least 72 h is often required to initiate CSII in newborns [21]. During hospitalization, parents must be properly instructed in bolus/basal insulin adjustments and management of potential CSII-related complications (including air bubbles, accidental infusion interruptions, and ketosis) [3, 18].

7.3.5 *Safety and Efficacy of CSII*

CSII efficacy has been well established in adults and its safety and feasibility have made it a well-accepted method for pediatric diabetes as well [43–45]. The safety and efficacy of CSII in NDM have also been supported. Park et al. showed stabilization of blood glucose values without hypoglycemia in newborns with NDM treated with a CSII [46]. However, there is currently no consensus on the use of CSII for the treatment of NDM.

7.4 SAP in NDM

There are three main components to SAP: a "smart" Insulin Pump, a CGM, and therapy management software. This combination has provided improvements in diabetes management as it presents additional benefits beyond those reached by CSII alone. By exploiting CGM threshold and trend alarms, SAP allows for prompt treatment of hyper- and hypoglycemia. Furthermore, predictive low glucose suspension algorithms provide an invaluable means of preventing hypoglycemia by suspending insulin delivery if CGM predicts glucose to fall according to predefined predictive thresholds. As a result, it is possible to optimize glucose control, thereby improving HbA1c and glucose variability, without increasing the risk of hypoglycemia [47].

The application of this technology is widespread among pediatric diabetes as suggested by the most recent international guidelines [2]. However, these devices are not approved in patients with NDM and only a few cases have been described in which CSII alone or SAP have been used.

An Italian study has shown the successful use of SAP applied in three cases of early-onset diabetes (including one SGA newborn) [17]. Two newborns were treated with the Animas Vibe pump (Animas Corp., West Chester, PA, USA) in combination with Dexcom G4 CG (Dexcom Inc., San Diego, CA, USA). In the first case, glucose excursions and insulin administration management improved. After having found mutations suggesting PNDM, insulin treatment was progressively shifted to oral sulfonylurea therapy, with further improvements in glucose control.

The second case also showed gradual improvement in glucose control and weight gain with a progressive reduction of insulin requirements. The infant was later diagnosed with transient NDM (TNDM).

The third case involved SAP use in a full-term female infant, born SGA and normoglycemic on the first day of life. At 24 days of life, she presented with irritability and failure to thrive. Routine blood tests showed hyperglycemia without ketoacidosis. A Minimed Paradigm Veo smart pump with Enlite sensor (Medtronic Inc., Minneapolis, MN, USA) was applied including low glucose threshold suspension (LGS) of insulin delivery. As this approach proved safe and effective, the baby (later diagnosed with PNDM) was discharged on SAP therapy.

The use of SAP in NDM is also reported in another study describing the case of a 3-month-old girl, presenting with irritability, lethargy, severe dehydration, and Kussmaul breathing patterns, associated with hyperglycemia and severe metabolic acidosis for which she was admitted to the PICU and treated with intravenous insulin infusion for 2 days until clinical stabilization. Genetic testing revealed a mutation in PNDM [48]. Therefore, a Minimed 530G system including an Enlite sensor and LGS (Medtronic, Inc., Northridge, CA) was applied. A Medtronic Sure-T insulin infusion set was used and changed every 2 weeks, while the sensor was applied to the baby's leg and changed every 6 days. Outpatient follow-up on SAP showed no sensor failures and no severe hypoglycemic events. HbA1c values progressively improved and adequate growth and age-appropriate milestones were achieved.

Finally, another Italian study described the use of SAP including LGS in a 1-month-old boy diagnosed with PNDM. In this case, the system was set with hypoglycemia alerts with a 2-h LGS of insulin delivery by the pump if glucose sensors detected a value under 80 mg/dL [16].

In the case of hyperglycemia, basal insulin infusion was increased by 0.025 units for every 100 mg/dL above the blood glucose value of 150 mg/dL. During the follow-up, no SAP-related adverse events were reported (including DKA or severe hypoglycemia) and glucose control improved.

Although few, the aforementioned cases support the efficacy, safety, and feasibility of CSII alone as well as SAP in the management of NDM. In particular, SAP systems may be superior to CSII alone in the prevention of severe hypoglycemic events, extreme glucose excursions, as CGM integration enables a more proactive and ever more accurate glucose control and management [1, 17]. Nonetheless, more studies are warranted before SAP may be confirmed in the routine clinical practice of NDM care.

7.5 Conclusion

In conclusion, clinical management of NDM is promising yet remains particularly challenging. There is an increasing interest in the use of technology in routine clinical practice, especially in newborns owing to their greater risk of complications (both hypoglycemia and hyperglycemia events which have been linked to adverse neurological outcomes) [49, 50]. Throughout an infant's growth, CSII therapy and CGM use in NDM needs to be carefully managed and supervised by a multidisciplinary team of neonatologists/pediatricians, nurses, dieticians, and psychologists experienced in the field of pediatric diabetes, who must also adequately educate and support the caregivers responsible for management at home. As there are currently limited clinical experiences and consensus guidelines are absent, the best therapeutic strategy in the management of NDM should therefore be tailored according to center-specific experience and the newborn's characteristics, with the ultimate objectives of achieving optimal glucose control, normal neurodevelopmental growth, and avoiding diabetes-related acute and long-term complications.

References

1. Rabbone I, Frontino G, Bonfanti R. Continuous subcutaneous insulin infusion and sensor-augmented pump therapy in children and adolescents. Diabetes Basel, Karger. 2015;24:143–50. https://doi.org/10.1159/000363488.
2. Sherr JL, Tauschmann M, Battelino T, de Bock M, Forlenza G, Roman R, et al. ISPAD clinical practice consensus guidelines 2018: diabetes technologies. Pediatr Diabetes. 2018;19:302–25. https://doi.org/10.1111/pedi.12731.
3. Bharucha T, Brown J, McDonnell C, Gebert R, McDougall P, Cameron F, et al. Neonatal diabetes mellitus: insulin pump as an alternative management strategy. J Paediatr Child Health. 2005;41:522–6. https://doi.org/10.1111/j.1440-1754.2005.00696.x.
4. Rabbone I. Tecnologia e categorie fragili. In: Diabete e tecnologia Terapia insulinica verso il futuro e oltre; 2018. p. 94.
5. Vettoretti M, Facchinetti A. Combining continuous glucose monitoring and insulin pumps to automatically tune the basal insulin infusion in diabetes therapy: a review. Biomed Eng Online. 2019;18:1–17. https://doi.org/10.1186/s12938-019-0658-x.
6. Baumeister F, Rolinski B, Busch R, Emmrich P. Glucose monitoring with long-term subcutaneous microdialysis in neonates. Pediatrics. 2001;108:1187–92. https://doi.org/10.1542/peds.108.5.1187.
7. McKinlay CJD, Alsweiler JM, Ansell JM, Anstice NS, Chase JG, Gamble GD, et al. Neonatal Glycemia and neurodevelopmental outcomes at 2 years. N Engl J Med. 2015;373:1507–18. https://doi.org/10.1056/NEJMoa1504909.
8. Galderisi A, Facchinetti A, Steil GM, Ortiz-Rubio P, Cavallin F, Tamborlane WV, et al. Continuous glucose monitoring in very preterm infants: a randomized controlled trial. Pediatrics. 2017;140:140. https://doi.org/10.1542/peds.2017-1162.
9. McKinlay CJD, Chase JG, Dickson J, Harris DL, Alsweiler JM, Harding JE. Continuous glucose monitoring in neonates: a review. Matern Heal Neonatol Perinatol. 2017;3:1–9. https://doi.org/10.1186/s40748-017-0055-z.
10. Rabbone I, Barbetti F, Gentilella R, Mossetto G, Bonfanti R, Maffeis C, et al. Insulin therapy in neonatal diabetes mellitus: a review of the literature. Diabetes Res Clin Pract. 2017;129:126–35. https://doi.org/10.1016/j.diabres.2017.04.007.
11. Basu SK, Kaiser JR, Guffey D, Minard CG, Guillet R, Gunn AJ. Hypoglycaemia and hyperglycaemia are associated with unfavourable outcome in infants with hypoxic ischaemic encephalopathy: a post hoc analysis of the CoolCap study. Arch Dis Child Fetal Neonatal Ed. 2016;101:F149–55. https://doi.org/10.1136/archdischild-2016-311385.
12. McKinlay CJD, Alsweiler JM, Anstice NS, Burakevych N, Chakraborty A, Chase JG, et al. Association of neonatal glycemia with neurodevelopmental outcomes at 4.5 years. JAMA Pediatr. 2017;171:972–83. https://doi.org/10.1001/jamapediatrics.2017.1579.
13. Mizumoto H, Kawai M, Yamashita S, Hata D. Intraday glucose fluctuation is common in preterm infants receiving intermittent tube feeding. Pediatr Int. 2016;58:359–62. https://doi.org/10.1111/ped.12838.
14. Beardsall K, Thomson L, Elleri D, Dunger DB, Hovorka R. Feasibility of automated insulin delivery guided by continuous glucose monitoring in preterm infants. Arch Dis Child Fetal Neonatal Ed. 2020;105:F279–84. https://doi.org/10.1136/archdischild-2019-316871.
15. Price G, Stevenson K, Walsh T. Evaluation of a continuous glucose monitor in an unselected general intensive care population. Crit Care Resusc. 2008;10:209–16.
16. Ortolani F, Piccinno E, Grasso V, Papadia F, Panzeca R, Cortese C, et al. Diabetes associated with dominant insulin gene mutations: outcome of 24-month, sensor-augmented insulin pump treatment. Acta Diabetol. 2016;53:499–501. https://doi.org/10.1007/s00592-015-0793-1.
17. Rabbone I, Barbetti F, Marigliano M, Bonfanti R, Piccinno E, Ortolani F, et al. Successful treatment of young infants presenting neonatal diabetes mellitus with continuous subcutaneous insulin infusion before genetic diagnosis. Acta Diabetol. 2016;53:559–65. https://doi.org/10.1007/s00592-015-0828-7.

18. Passanisi S, Timpanaro T, Lo Presti D, Mammì C, Caruso-Nicoletti M. Treatment of transient neonatal diabetes mellitus: insulin pump or insulin glargine? Our experience. Diabetes Technol Ther. 2014;16:880–4. https://doi.org/10.1089/dia.2014.0055.
19. Phillip M, Danne T, Shalitin S, Buckingham B, Laffel L, Tamborlane W, et al. Use of continuous glucose monitoring in children and adolescents. Pediatr Diabetes. 2012;13:215–28. https://doi.org/10.1111/j.1399-5448.2011.00849.x.
20. Lemelman MB, Letourneau L, Greeley SAW. Neonatal diabetes mellitus: an update on diagnosis and management. Clin Perinatol. 2018;45:41–59. https://doi.org/10.1016/j.clp.2017.10.006.
21. Bonfanti R, et al. Raccomandazioni sull'utilizzo della tecnologia in diabetologia pediatrica 2019. Acta Biomed. 2019;90(1):5–88.
22. Karges B, Meissner T, Icks A, Kapellen T, Holl RW. Management of diabetes mellitus in infants. Nat Rev Endocrinol. 2011;8:201–11. https://doi.org/10.1038/nrendo.2011.204.
23. Rabbone I, Barbetti F, Gentilella R, Mossetto G, Bonfanti R, Maffeis C, et al. Insulin therapy in neonatal diabetes mellitus. Diabetes Res Clin Pract. 2017;129:126–35. https://doi.org/10.1016/j.diabres.2017.04.007.
24. Novo Nordisk Limited. NovoRapid PumpCart 100 units/ml: summary of product characteristics. Gatwick UNNLJ; 2015.
25. Sanofi. Apidra 100 units/ml, solution for injection in a cartridge: summary of product characteristics. Guildford US 24 O 2013.
26. Noble SL, Johnston E, Walton B. Insulin lispro: a fast-acting insulin analog. Am Fam Physician. 1998;57(279–286):289–92.
27. Eli Lilly and Company Limited. Humalog 100U/ml, solution for injection in vial, Humalog 100U/ml, solution for injection in Cartridge, Humalog KwikPen 100U/ml, solution for injection: summary of product characteristics. Basingstoke UEL and CL 23 A 2014.
28. Pozzilli P, Battelino T, Danne T, Hovorka R, Jarosz-Chobot P, Renard E. Continuous subcutaneous insulin infusion in diabetes: patient populations, safety, efficacy, and pharmacoeconomics. Diabetes Metab Res Rev. 2016;32:21–39. https://doi.org/10.1002/dmrr.2653.
29. Olinder AL, Kernell A, Smide B. Treatment with CSII in two infants with neonatal diabetes mellitus. Pediatr Diabetes. 2006;7:284–8. https://doi.org/10.1111/j.1399-5448.2006.00203.x.
30. Beardsall K, Pesterfield CL, Acerini CL. Neonatal diabetes and insulin pump therapy. Arch Dis Child Fetal Neonatal Ed. 2011;96:223–5. https://doi.org/10.1136/adc.2010.196709.
31. Danne T, Bangstad H-J, Deeb L, Jarosz-Chobot P, Mungaie L, Saboo B, et al. ISPAD clinical practice consensus guidelines 2014. Insulin treatment in children and adolescents with diabetes. Pediatr Diabetes. 2014 Sep;15(Suppl 2):115–34. https://doi.org/10.1111/pedi.12184.
32. Ortolani F, Tummolo A, Grasso V, Papadia F, Vendemiale M, Masciopinto M, et al. Neonatal permanent diabetes caused by mutation INS/Y50C: integrated system CGMS and insulin pump [poster]. ICE/ENDO 2014, Chicago 2014 June 22.
33. Kapellen TM, Heidtmann B, Lilienthal E, Rami-Merhar B, Engler-Schmidt C, Holl RW. Continuous subcutaneous insulin infusion in neonates and infants below 1 year: analysis of initial bolus and basal rate based on the experiences from the German working group for pediatric pump treatment. Diabetes Technol Ther. 2015;17:872–9. https://doi.org/10.1089/dia.2015.0030.
34. Barbetti F, D'Annunzio G. Genetic causes and treatment of neonatal diabetes and early childhood diabetes. Best Pract Res Clin Endocrinol Metab. 2018;32:575–91. https://doi.org/10.1016/j.beem.2018.06.008.
35. Tubiana-Rufi N. Insulin pump therapy in neonatal diabetes. In: Development of the pancreas and neonatal diabetes. Basel: KARGER; 2007. p. 67–74.
36. Wintergerst KA, Hargadon S, Hsiang HY. Continuous subcutaneous insulin infusion in neonatal diabetes mellitus. Pediatr Diabetes. 2004;5:202–6. https://doi.org/10.1111/j.1399-543X.2004.00067.x.
37. Pickup JC. Management of diabetes mellitus: is the pump mightier than the pen? Nat Rev Endocrinol. 2012;8:425–33. https://doi.org/10.1038/nrendo.2012.28.

38. Fendler W, Baranowska AI, Mianowska B, Szadkowska A, Mlynarski W. Three-year comparison of subcutaneous insulin pump treatment with multi-daily injections on HbA1c, its variability and hospital burden of children with type 1 diabetes. Acta Diabetol. 2012;49:363–70. https://doi.org/10.1007/s00592-011-0332-7.
39. Levy-Shraga Y, Lerner-Geva L, Modan-Moses D, Graph-Barel C, Mazor-Aronovitch K, Boyko V, et al. Benefits of continuous subcutaneous insulin infusion (CSII) therapy in preschool children. Exp Clin Endocrinol diabetes Off journal, Ger Soc Endocrinol [and] Ger Diabetes Assoc. 2013;121:225–9. https://doi.org/10.1055/s-0032-1331698.
40. Alyafie F, Soliman AT, Sabt A, Elawwa A, Alkhalaf F, Alzyoud M, et al. Postnatal growth of infants with neonatal diabetes: insulin pump (CSII) versus multiple daily injection (MDI) therapy. Acta Biomed. 2019;90:28–35. https://doi.org/10.23750/abm.v90i8-S.6719.
41. Pinelli L, Rabbone I, Salardi S, Toni S, Scaramuzza A, Bonfanti R, et al. Insulin pump therapy in children and adolescents with type 1 diabetes: the Italian viewpoint. Acta Biomed. 2008;79:57–64.
42. Ross PL, Milburn J, Reith DM, Wiltshire E, Wheeler BJ. Clinical review: insulin pump-associated adverse events in adults and children. Vol. 52, Acta Diabetologica. Springer-Verlag Italia s.r.l; 2015. p. 1017–24.
43. Phillip M, Battelino T, Rodriguez H, Danne T, Kaufman F. Use of insulin pump therapy in the pediatric age-group: consensus statement from the European society for Paediatric endocrinology, the Lawson Wilkins pediatric endocrine society, and the international society for pediatric and adolescent diabetes, endors. Diabetes Care. 2007;30:1653–62. https://doi.org/10.2337/dc07-9922.
44. Weinzimer SA, Swan KL, Sikes KA, Ahern JH. Emerging evidence for the use of insulin pump therapy in infants, toddlers, and preschool-aged children with type 1 diabetes. Pediatr Diabetes. 2006;7(Suppl 4):15–9. https://doi.org/10.1111/j.1399-543X.2006.00172.x.
45. Mecklenburg RS, Benson EA, Benson JWJ, Blumenstein BA, Fredlund PN, Guinn TS, et al. Long-term metabolic control with insulin pump therapy. Report of experience with 127 patients. N Engl J Med. 1985;313:465–8. https://doi.org/10.1056/NEJM198508223130802.
46. Park JH, Kang JH, Lee K-H, Kim N-H, Yoo H-W, Lee D-Y, et al. Insulin pump therapy in transient neonatal diabetes mellitus. Ann Pediatr Endocrinol Metab. 2013;18:148. https://doi.org/10.6065/apem.2013.18.3.148.
47. Nicolucci A, Rossi MC, D'Ostilio D, Delbaere A, de Portu S, Roze S. Cost-effectiveness of sensor-augmented pump therapy in two different patient populations with type 1 diabetes in Italy. Nutr Metab Cardiovasc Dis. 2018 Jul;28(7):707–15.
48. Marin MT, Coffey ML, Beck JK, Dasari PS, Allen R, Krishnan S. A novel approach to the management of neonatal diabetes using sensor-augmented insulin pump therapy with threshold suspend technology at diagnosis. Diabetes Spectr. 2016;29:176–9. https://doi.org/10.2337/diaspect.29.3.176.
49. Northam EA, Anderson PJ, Jacobs R, Hughes M, Warne GL, Werther GA. Neuropsychological profiles of children with type 1 diabetes 6 years after disease onset. Diabetes Care. 2001;2001(24):1541–6. https://doi.org/10.2337/diacare.24.9.1541.
50. Ferguson SC, Blane A, Wardlaw J, Frier BM, Perros P, McCrimmon RJ, et al. Influence of an early-onset age of type 1 diabetes on cerebral structure and cognitive function. Diabetes Care. 2005;28:1431–7. https://doi.org/10.2337/diacare.28.6.1431.

Chapter 8
Oral Pharmacological Treatment of Neonatal Diabetes

Dario Iafusco, Angela Zanfardino, Alessia Piscopo, and Emanuele Miraglia del Giudice

Abbreviations

CGM	Continuous Glucose Monitoring
SAP	Sensor Augmented Pump
PNDM	Permanent Neonatal Diabetes Mellitus
TNDM	Transient Neonatal Diabetes Mellitus
K_{ATP}	ATP-sensitive K^{+}-channel
OHA	Oral Hypoglycemic Agents
DKA	Diabetes ketoacidosis

Shortly after the diagnosis of neonatal diabetes, the choice of insulin treatment (intravenous insulin therapy, subcutaneously by pens or by pump) must be customized according to the clinical condition of the newborn [1]. As reported in the paragraph on insulin therapy, it is useful to choose pumps that deliver very small doses of insulin to obviate the need for drug dilution [2]. Horizontal cannulas are less likely than perpendicular cannulas to penetrate deeper than the subcutaneous tissue, a significant issue for infants in whom subcutaneous fat quantities may be marginal

Supplementary Information The online version contains supplementary material available at https://doi.org/10.1007/978-3-031-07008-2_8.

D. Iafusco (✉) · A. Zanfardino · A. Piscopo · E. M. del Giudice
Department of Woman, Child, and General and Specia listic Surgery, University of Campania "Luigi Vanvitelli", Regional Centre of Pediatric Diabetology "G.Stoppoloni", Naples, Italy
e-mail: dario.iafusco@unicampania.it; angela.zanfardino@unicampania.it; alessia.piscopo@policliniconapoli.it; emanuele.miragliadelgiudice@unicampania.it

I. Rabbone, D. Iafusco (eds.), *Neonatal and Early Onset Diabetes Mellitus*, https://doi.org/10.1007/978-3-031-07008-2_8

for cannula insertion [3]. Some evidences indicate better glycemic control in small children receiving insulin pump therapy when infusion set is inserted in the buttock rather than the abdomen [4]. Continuous Glucose Monitoring (CGM) is used to improve glucose monitoring in newborns at risk of fluctuating glucose levels, particularly hypoglycemia [5]. In particular Sensor Augmenting Pumps (SAP) therapy has proven to be safe and effective in treating neonatal diabetes at the onset and in switching from insulin to Glibenclamide therapy in Permanent Neonatal Diabetes Mellitus (PNDM) [6].

Most patients with activating mutations in KCNJ11 or ABCC8 can be successfully switched from insulin to oral sulfonylurea, with a marked improvement in metabolic control [7].

Mutations in the Kir6.2 subunit of the ATP-sensitive potassium channel (K_{ATP}) or mutations in sulfonylurea (SU) receptors (SURs) underlie neonatal diabetes mellitus because disruption of K_{ATP} activity impairs insulin release and results in inappropriate serum insulin levels.

In pancreatic β-cell, the ATP-sensitive K^+-channel (K_{ATP}) regulates insulin secretion by coupling changes in metabolism (represented by the concentration ratio of ATP to ADP) with changes in electrical activity. In normal people, as blood glucose levels rise, the intracellular ATP to ADP ratio increases causing, in succession, closure of K_{ATP} channels, membrane depolarization, voltage-driven influx of Ca^{2+}, and Ca^{2+}-dependent insulin release [8].

The mature K_{ATP} channel exists as a hetero-octomer of four pore-forming Kir6.2 subunits (*KCNJ11* gene) and four regulatory sulfonylurea receptors (*ABCC8* gene). The Kir6.2 subunit contains the binding site for inhibitory ATP, whereas the SUR subunit confers channel stimulation by Mg nucleotides and inhibition to SU drugs. With respect to SU block, an added level of complexity arises from the existence of multiple SUR isoforms (SUR1, SUR2A, and SUR2B), which exhibit differential tissue expression and SU sensitivities [9].

Specifically, heterozygous activating mutations in K_{ATP} (both the Kir6.2 and the SUR1 subunits) are causal both in permanent (PNDM) and in transient (TNDM) forms of neonatal diabetes mellitus in humans. In approximately one-third of the cases, K_{ATP} mutations are associated with developmental delay (both motor and intellectual), epilepsy, and neonatal diabetes (DEND syndrome), and extrapancreatic symptoms are likely the result of overactive K_{ATP} in muscle, peripheral nerves, and/or brain. In intermediate DEND the patient with neonatal diabetes exhibits developmental delay but not epilepsy, and in most cases, this form of DEND is associated with the V59M mutation.

Sulfonylureas, by binding to the sulfonylurea receptor, can close the KATP channel. This has led to patients who were insulin-dependent being able to discontinue insulin injections and achieve excellent control with sulfonylurea tablets [10].

For this reason, sulfonylurea (SU) compounds that specifically inhibit K_{ATP} and thereby stimulate insulin secretion have proven a valuable alternative to insulin therapy in treating hyperglycemia in patients with activating K_{ATP} mutations [11].

Also, the skeletal muscle K_{ATP} (Kir6.2 + SUR2A) channel is sensitive to glibenclamide, although the success rate seems to be lower in patients with DEND symptoms.

The required doses of sulfonylurea are usually high, especially in patients with neurological features, but tend to decrease over time irrespective of the mutation [12].

In the European cohort of 81 patients with Neonatal Diabetes by KCNJ11 mutation the median sulfonylurea dose was 0,3 mg/kg per day (0,14-0,53 mg/Kg/day) at 1 year and at most recent follow-up visit after 12 years was 0,23 mg/kg/day (0,12–0,41 mg/Kg/day) [13]. A maximal dose of sulfonylurea for treating patients with K_{ATP} mutations has not been established. No reports of severe hypoglycemia were reported in 809 patient years of follow up for the whole cohort.

Very intriguing are the demonstrations of the different affinity and organ specificity of the first respect to the second generation sulfonylureas. The sulfonylurea of first generation, as Glibenclamide, exerts its action not only on the beta cell but also on neuromuscular junctions and heart tissue while the more recent gliclazide acts specifically on insulin secretion only.

Koster, Cadario et al. described an adult with intermediate DEND with heterozygous mutation in Kir6.2 (G53D) weaned from insulin into gliclazide and then glibenclamide, resulting in good glycemic control, although gliclazide treatment required supplemental insulin. Importantly, motor features were improved only by glibenclamide as assessed by increased muscle coordination and an enhanced gait [8].

The timing of switch from insulin to Glibenclamide therapy in Permanent Neonatal Diabetes Mellitus (PNDM) is actually discussed. Sulfonylurea therapy can improve glycemic control and ameliorate neurodevelopmental outcomes in patients suffering from Neonatal Diabetes Mellitus (NDM) with KCNJ11 or ABCC8 mutations. As genetic testing results are often delayed, it remains controversial whether sulfonylurea treatment should be attempted immediately after the diagnosis or whether doctors should await genetic confirmation [14].

Recently, we have reported the case of an infant born small for gestational age (SGA; 2100 g, <3rd centile), the daughter of a PNDM patient carrying the *KCNJ11* mutation R201C, was diagnosed with neonatal diabetes right after birth (blood glucose fluctuating between 4.4 and 22.2 mmol/l (80 and 400 mg/dl). The markers of autoimmune diabetes (autoantibodies to GAD, islet antigen 2 [IA2], and zinc transporter 8 [ZnT8] and insulin autoantibodies [IAA]) were negative. Family history prompted us to commence treatment with the sulfonylurea glibenclamide at a dose of 0.36 mg kg^{-1} day^{-1} (in three administrations) on day 3 of life, before the report confirming that she had inherited the paternal mutation (obtained at 12 days of life). However, because of a failure to thrive (steadily decreasing body weight, down to 1950 g) and unsatisfactory metabolic control, insulin was added to sulfonylureas for about a month, resulting in the patient's weight gain of approximately 180 g per week. At 42 days of life, she was finally weaned from insulin injections at the glibenclamide dose of 0.92 mg kg^{-1} day^{-1}.

For this reason, also if some outcomes suggest that functional β-cells may be preserved with low doses of sulfonylurea started very early in life without insulin administration or risk of severe hypoglycemia [15]. This is consistent with murine data indicating that early treatment with sulfonylureas preserves β-cells in K_{ATP}-dependent diabetes [16], we think that it could not be a good idea in newborns with diabetes with the suspect of mutation of the channel of potassium born small for gestational age to start the glibenclamide as soon after the birth in order to make it grow thanks to insulin therapy just enough to start immediately after the treatment with oral hypoglycemic.

Oral Hypoglycemic Agents (OHA) side effects in neonatal diabetes are definitely less than the benefits. Diarrhea during sulfonylurea treatment in neonates is transient and usually does not require interruption of therapy. Staining of the teeth has been noted in the longer-term treated patients [17].

Following transfer to sulfonylureas, was noted improvement of nervous system impairment in patients with CNS features.

During the treatment with oral agents in patients with *KCNJ11* or *SUR-1* mutation it is mandatory that the absorption of the drug is effective.

In the case reported by us, she remained in good metabolic control for 3 years, with HbA_{1c} below 42 mmol/mol (6%) at every trimestral visit. At 38 months of age (June 2016), she presented with fever, vomiting, and biochemical evidence of Diabetic Ketoacidosis (DKA): arterial pH 7.1, blood glucose 22.2 mmol/l (400 mg/dl), ketonemia 6 mmol/l, in the presence of a relative decrease of body weight that occurred a few months before the onset of hyperglycemia. HbA_{1c} 6 months before and at the time of the DKA episode was normal (37 mmol/mol [5.5%]. Glibenclamide (dose at the time of hospitalization: 0.08 mg kg^{-1} day^{-1}) was stopped and insulin therapy was commenced according to the Glucose Evaluation Trial for Remission (GETREM) protocol (0.05 U kg^{-1} day^{-1} i.v.) [18]. The parents informed us that there had been no changes in the therapeutic regimen and so we sought the possible causes of metabolic derangement.

Further investigations revealed that the patient carried coeliac disease-predisposing HLA haplotypes (HLA DQ2 positive, DQ8 negative) and unequivocally elevated Transglutaminase 2 (TG2) IgA (96 U/ml; positive >16 U/ml). Jejunal biopsy confirmed the diagnosis of coeliac disease. A gluten-free diet was prescribed to the patient with normalization of aminotransferases, blood iron levels and erythrocyte analysis, and a substantial decrease of TG2 IgA titer (7.0 U/ml after 1 year; negative <9 U/ml), a sign of adherence to the gluten-free diet [6]. Six months from the start of the gluten-free diet, glibenclamide was reintroduced at the same dose (i.e., 0.08 mg kg^{-1} day^{-1}) that was administered at the time of hospitalization (Fig. 8.1.). Over a period of about 3 years glibenclamide was progressively tapered off to the current dose of 0.04 mg kg^{-1} day^{-1}. HbA_{1c} remained stable between 39 and 40 mmol/mol [5.8–5.9%], slightly higher than the values observed immediately before and during insulin therapy for DKA.

Data collected by the Italian Group of Study of Diabetes of Italian Society of Pediatric Endocrinology and Diabetology (ISPED) on the long-term consequences of diabetes with onset in the neonatal period are very intriguing [19]. They have

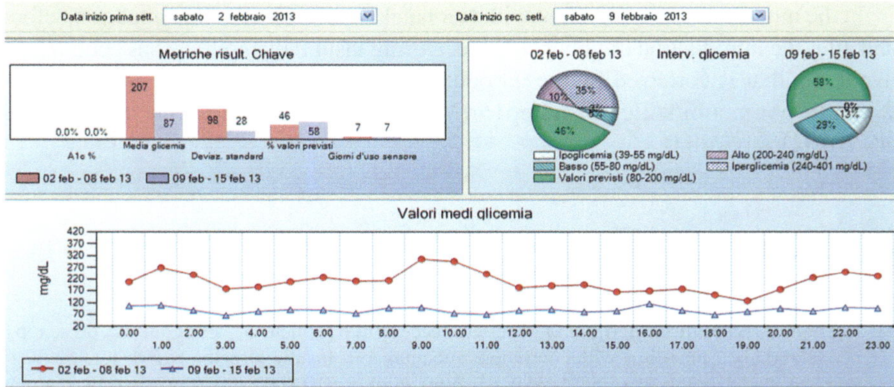

Fig. 8.1. This picture shows the different metabolic control in an infant with permanent neonatal diabetes during insulin (red dots) or glibenclamide (blue triangles) therapy (personal observation)

demonstrated that the impact of long-standing diabetes (more than 15 years) on the retina is very little compared with diabetes onset in other ages. Proliferative retinopathy was reported in none of 10 patients with neonatal diabetes. Fifty-three percent of patients with diabetes duration between 16 and 24 years had no sign of diabetic retinopathy, 33% were judged to have mild retinopathy and 7% had moderate diabetic retinopathy with possible initial signs of diabetic macular edema and only 7% had diabetic macular edema. All patients with mild or moderate diabetic retinopathy had diabetes for more than 30 years but one.

In the European cohort with alteration of KIR6.2, seven (9%) patients had microvascular complications; these patients had been taking insulin longer than those without complications (median age at transfer from insulin to sulfonylureas 20,5 years (IQR 10,5–24,0) vs 4,1 years (1,3–10,2); $p = 0.0005$) [20]. Hypoglycemic episodes also appear to be rare in patients treated with Glibenclamide differently from what happens in children with Type 1 Diabetes treated with insulin.[7]

The debate is particularly open on the type of therapy to recommend to patients with recurrent transient neonatal diabetes at the time of recurrence of disease at the time of puberty or in the young adult. The most common pathogenesis of these forms is due to the isodisomia of chromosome 6q that involves an increase of action of two apoptotic genes: ZAC and Hymai which involve beta cellular apoptosis. In addition, the HYMAI gene is also involved in insulin secretion [21].

To avoid insulin therapy at the time of recurrence of the disease it was tried to use sulfonylureas. Recently, we have used gliclazide with little success (Iafusco et al. personal communication). Many Authors have reported the role of noninsulin therapies alone or in combination in chromosome 6q24-related transient neonatal diabetes: Sulfonylurea improves but does not always normalize insulin secretion; whereas there is also the anecdotical experience of relapsing 6q24-related transient neonatal diabetes mellitus successfully treated with a dipeptidyl peptidase-4 inhibitor [22].

In the movie, we show an infant with Neonatal Diabetes by KIR6.2 mutation before and after the introduction of glibenclamide. During insulin therapy, she has generalized hypotonia that is corrected by the introduction of Oral Hypoglycemic Drug. https://www.dropbox.com/s/2lectdnrv2pp16r/Mutation%20KIR%20Iafusco%20et%20al%202021.mpg?dl=0

References

1. Rabbone I, Barbetti F, Marigliano M, et al. Successful treatment of young infants presenting neonatal diabetes mellitus with continuous subcutaneous insulin infusion before genetic diagnosis. Acta Diabetol. 2016;53(4):559–65. https://doi.org/10.1007/s00592-015-0828-7. Epub 2016 Feb 1
2. Olinder AL, Kernell A, Smide B. Treatment with CSII in two infants with neonatal diabetes mellitus. Pediatr Diabetes. 2006;7(5):284–8.
3. Rabbone I, Barbetti F, Gentilella R, Mossetto G, Bonfanti R, Maffeis C, Iafusco D, Piccinno E. Insulin therapy in neonatal diabetes mellitus: a review of the literature. Diabetes Res Clin Pract. 2017;129:126–35. https://doi.org/10.1016/j.diabres.2017.04.007. Epub 2017 Apr 13
4. Zanfardino A, Iafusco D, Piscopo A, Cocca A, Villano P, Confetto S, Caredda E, Picariello S, Russo L, Casaburo F, Rollato AS, Forgione E, Zuccotti G, Prisco F, Scaramuzza AE. Continuous subcutaneous insulin infusion in preschool children: butt or tummy, which is the best infusion set site? Diabetes Technol Ther. 2014;16(9):563–6. https://doi.org/10.1089/dia.2013.0357. Epub 2014 May 6
5. Rabbone I, Barbetti F, Gentilella R, et al. Insulin therapy in neonatal diabetes mellitus: a review of the literature. Diabetes Res Clin Pract. 2017;129:126–35. https://doi.org/10.1016/j.diabres.2017.04.007. Epub 2017 Apr 13
6. Ortolani F, Piccinno E, Grasso V, et al. Diabetes associated with dominant insulin gene mutations: outcome of 24 month, sensor augmented insulin pump treatment. Acta Diabetol. 2016;53(3):499–501. https://doi.org/10.1007/s00592-015-0793-1. Epub 2015 Aug 4
7. Iafusco D, Zanfardino A, Bonfanti R, Rabbone I, Tinto N, Iafusco F, Meola S, Gicchino MF, Ozen G, Casaburo F, Piscopo A, Miraglia Del Giudice E, Barbetti F. Congenital diabetes mellitus. Minerva Pediatr. 2020;72(4):240–9. https://doi.org/10.23736/S0026-4946.20.05838-7. Epub 2020 Apr 9.
8. Koster JC, Cadario F, Peruzzi C, Colombo C, Nichols CG, Barbetti F. The G53D mutation in Kir6.2 (KCNJ11) is associated with neonatal diabetes and motor dysfunction in adulthood that is improved with sulfonylurea therapy. J Clin Endocrinol Metab. 2008;93(3):1054–61. https://doi.org/10.1210/jc.2007-1826. Epub 2007 Dec 11
9. Gribble FM, Tucker SJ. Ashcroft FM The interaction of nucleotides with the tolbutamide block of cloned ATP-sensitive K+ channel currents expressed in Xenopus oocytes: a reinterpretation. J Physiol. 1997;504:35–45.
10. Slingerland AS. Hattersley AT Mutations in the Kir6.2 subunit of the KATP channel and permanent neonatal diabetes: new insights and new treatment. Ann Med. 2005;37(3):186–95. https://doi.org/10.1080/07853890510007287.
11. Pearson ER, Flechtner I, Njolstad PR, Malecki MT, Flanagan SE, Larkin B, Ashcroft FM, Klimes I, Codner E, Iotova V, Slingerland AS, Shield J, Robert JJ, Holst JJ, Clark PM, Ellard S, Sovik O, Polak M, Hattersley AT. Switching from insulin to oral sulfonylureas in patients with diabetes due to Kir6.2 mutations. N Engl J Med. 2006;355:467–77.
12. Massa O, Iafusco D, D'Amato E, Gloyn AL, Hattersley AT, Pasquino B, Tonini G, Dammacco F, Zanette G, Meschi F, Porzio O, Bottazzo G, Crinó A, Lorini R, Cerutti F, Vanelli M, Barbetti F. KCNJ11 activating mutations in Italian patients with permanent neonatal diabetes. Early

onset diabetes study group of the Italian Society of Pediatric Endocrinology and Diabetology. Hum Mutat. 2005 Jan;25(1):22–7. https://doi.org/10.1002/humu.20124.

13. Bowman P, Sulen Å, Barbetti F, Beltrand J, Svalastoga P, Codner E, Tessmann EH, Juliusson PB, Skrivarhaug T, Pearson ER, Flanagan SE, Babiker T, Thomas NJ, Shepherd MH, Ellard S, Klimes I, Szopa M, Polak M, Iafusco D, Hattersley AT, Njølstad PR. Neonatal Diabetes International Collaborative Group. Effectiveness and safety of longterm treatment with sulfonylureas in patients with neonatal diabetes due to KCNJ11 mutations: an international cohort study. Lancet Diabetes Endocrinol. 2018;6(8):637–46. https://doi.org/10.1016/S2213-8587(18)30106-2. Epub 2018
14. Li X, Aijing X, Sheng H, Ting TH, Mao X, Huamg X, Jiang M, Cheng J, Liu L. Early transition from insulin to sulfonylureas in neonatal diabetes and follow-up: experience from China. Pediatr Diabetes. 2018;19(2):251–8. https://doi.org/10.1111/pedi.12560. Epub 2017 Aug 8
15. Marshall BA, Green RP, Wambach J, Whiate NH. Remedi MS and Nichols CG remission of severe neonatal diabetes with very early sulfonylurea treatment. Diabetes Care. 2015 Mar;38(3):e38–9.
16. Remedi MS, Agapova SE, Vyas AK, Hruz PW, Nichols CG. Acute sulfonylurea therapy at disease onset can cause permanent remission of KATP-induced diabetes. Diabetes. 2011;60:2515–22.
17. Kumaraguru J, Flanagan SE, Greeley SA, Nuboer R, Støy J, Philipson LH, Hattersley AT, Rubio-Cabezas O. Tooth discoloration in patients with neonatal diabetes after transfer onto glibenclamide: a previously unreported side effect. Diabetes Care. 2009;32:1428–30. https://doi.org/10.2337/dc09-0280. Epub 2009 May 12
18. Pozzilli P, Manfrini S, Buzzetti R, Lampeter E, De Leeuw I, Iafusco D, Prisco F, Ionescu-Tirgoviste C, Kolouskovà S, Linn T, Ludvigsson J, Madàcsy L, Seremak Mrozikiewicz A, Mrozikiewicz PM, Podar T, Vavrinec J, Vialettes B, Visalli N, Yilmaz T, Browne PD. IMDIAB Group Glucose evaluation trial for remission (GETREM) in type 1 diabetes: a European multicentre study. Diabetes Res Clin Pract. 2005;68(3):258–64. https://doi.org/10.1016/j.diabres.2004.10.001. Epub 2004 Nov 21
19. Iafusco D, Salardi S, Chiari G, et al. Early onset diabetes study group of the Italian Society of Pediatric Endocrinology and Diabetology (ISPED). No sign of proliferative retinopathy in 15 patients with permanent neonatal diabetes with a median diabetes duration of 24 years. Diabetes Care. 2014; Aug;37(8):e181–2. https://doi.org/10.2337/dc14-0471.
20. Flechtner I, de Lonlay P, Polak M. Diabetes and hypoglycaemia in young children and mutations in the Kir6.2 subunit of the potassium channel: therapeutic consequences. Diabetes Metab. 2006; Dec;32(6):569–80.
21. Carmody D, Beca FA, Bell CD, Hwang JL, Dickens JT, Devine NA, Mackay DJG, Temple IK, Hays LR, Naylor RN, Philipson LH. Greeley SAW Role of noninsulin therapies alone or in combination in chromosome 6q24-Related transient neonatal diabetes: sulfonylurea improves but does not always normalize insulin secretion. Diabetes Care. 2015;38:e86–7.
22. Yorifuji T, Hashimoto Y, Kawakita R, Hosokawa Y, Fujimaru R, Hatake K, Tamagawa N, Nakajima H. Fujii M Relapsing 6q24-related transient neonatal diabetes mellitus successfully treated with a dipeptidyl peptidase-4 inhibitor: a case report. Pediatr Diabetes. 2014;15:606–10.

Chapter 9
Complications Acute and Chronic

Marco Marigliano, Alberto Sabbion, Giovanna Contreas, and Claudio Maffeis

9.1 Gene Mutations

9.1.1 HNF4A

Hepatocyte nuclear factor-4-alpha (HNF4A) is a DNA-binding protein that is found in abundance in the liver, where it regulates genes involved in lipid metabolism and hepatic gluconeogenesis. Mutations in the HNF4A gene cause a reduction in insulin secretion.

The clinical presentation related to HNF4A mutation (MODY1) is characterized by a steady increase in blood glucose over time. The beta-cell response is decreased as insulin secretion is impaired by the defect in the transcription factor. Due to progressive worsening of blood glucose control, these patients may present the full spectrum of diabetes complications. Microvascular complications, in particular, those involving the retina and kidneys, are as common as in patients with Type 1 or Type 2 diabetes and are related to overall glycemic control [1, 2].

Supplementary Information The online version contains supplementary material available at https://doi.org/10.1007/978-3-031-07008-2_9.

M. Marigliano · A. Sabbion · G. Contreas · C. Maffeis (✉)
Pediatric Diabetes and Metabolic Disorders Unit, University of Verona, Verona, Italy
e-mail: marco.marigliano@univr.it; claudio.maffeis@univr.it

I. Rabbone, D. Iafusco (eds.), *Neonatal and Early Onset Diabetes Mellitus*, https://doi.org/10.1007/978-3-031-07008-2_9

9.1.2 Glucokinase

Glucokinase (GCK) is a hexokinase that regulates the first step in glycolysis, converting glucose into glucose-6 phosphate. This enzyme has unique functional characteristics and plays a pivotal role in the regulation of glucose metabolism. The MODY GCK-related is characterized by mild nonprogressive hyperglycemia and is often misdiagnosed as Type 2 diabetes, representing a possible cause of *gestational-like* diabetes [3].

Patients with GCK mutations are characterized by a particularly low rate of vascular complications, substantially less than those associated with other forms of diabetes [4, 5]. The reported prevalence of clinically significant microvascular complications (background retinopathy or persistent microalbuminuria or proteinuria) was 1%, which did not differ from the percentage detected in the healthy controls. In this same cohort, about one-third of patients with GCK mutations had background retinopathy as compared to 14% of the healthy controls. No severe eye complications were described. Microalbuminuria and neuropathies were equally frequent as in the control population, the rate of macrovascular complications was lower than in healthy subjects [5].

9.1.3 Hepatocyte Nuclear Factor-1-Alpha

Hepatocyte nuclear factor-1-alpha (HNF1A) is a transcription factor required for the expression of several liver-specific genes. Mutations in the HNF1A gene can cause deregulation of the molecular mechanisms and lead to diabetes mellitus.

The glycemic pattern in patients with HNF1A mutations is characterized by mild fasting hyperglycemia and very high glucose concentrations following glucose administration [6]. The renal glucose threshold is lower in patients with HNF1A mutations than in the healthy population. These patients may have the full spectrum of micro- and macrovascular complications, involving both the retina and the kidneys, at a similar frequency as in patients with Type 1 and Type 2 diabetes. The development of such complications is related to the level of metabolic control [1, 6, 7].

9.1.4 HNF1B

Renal cysts and diabetes syndrome (RCAD) occur more frequently in isolated cases due to the de novo origin of the HNF1B mutations. Differently from the other subtypes of monogenic diabetes, large genomic rearrangements, and gene deletions occurred in HNF1B–MODY cases [8, 9]. Onset occurs typically during adolescence or early adulthood even if neonatal onset has also been reported. There is little mention of chronic complications in literature but they may be as common as in other types of diabetes and related to glycemic control [10].

9.1.5 KCNJ11 and ABCC8

Mutations in the KCNJ11 gene encoding the pore-forming subunit of the ATP-dependent potassium channel (KATP) (KIR6.2) and in the ABCC8 gene encoding its regulatory subunit (SUR1) are among the most common causes of neonatal diabetes. For the former, the most common form is permanent, while the latter is more frequently a form of transient neonatal diabetes [11]. The neurological involvement often found in infants with mutations in the KCNJ11 and ABCC8 genes can be aggravated by improper treatment that does not allow adequate glycemic control, essential for regular neurological development [12, 13]. Over 95% of subjects with mutations in the genes of the KATP channel respond to treatment with sulfonylurea (SU), which is usually well tolerated: only occasionally it can cause diarrhea that can be resolved in most cases without stopping the intake. Most of these patients are misdiagnosed as having other types of diabetes and erroneously treated with insulin, which may result in poor control and episodes of hypoglycemia.

The efficacy and safety of this treatment were also excellent in the long term, as recently reported in a cohort of 81 patients with KCNJ11 gene mutations, 93% of whom were not taking insulin after 10 years of SU therapy [14]. In this large cohort, the authors found low rates of diabetes-related microvascular complications and no hypoglycemic episodes or weight gain were found in SU-treated patients, suggesting finely regulated endogenous insulin secretion.

The development of complications in seven (9%) patients was attributed to the suboptimal glycemic control shown in the years prior to initiation of SU therapy, which occurred at an older age than in other uncomplicated subjects (median 20.5 years versus 4.1 years). In contrast to the excellent glycemic response, the effect of SU on neurological functions, after some initial improvements, was usually incomplete.

Furthermore, the incidence of psychiatric disorders (ADHD, autism, anxiety, and mood disorders) was higher than in the pediatric reference population and with association with the V59M and R201C mutations of the KCNJ11 gene [15, 16].

While these disorders have a significant impact on families, they may be clinically underestimated [5]. For these reasons, careful neurological follow-up and a multidisciplinary approach to the complex needs of these patients are advisable [16].

9.1.6 Insulin

For neonatal diabetes resulting from the mutation of the insulin gene (INS), lacking an involvement of other organs and for similarity with Type 1 diabetes mellitus, we can consider that the acute (severe hypoglycemia and ketoacidosis) and chronic (microvascular complications) complications, will be closely related to insulin therapy and the level of glycometabolic control obtained.

However, it should be noted that in the studies where patients with age of onset of Type 1 diabetes in the first years of life were examined, the results showed a protective effect of young age against the development of diabetic retinopathy compared to a later diagnosis [17, 18]; this advantage that can, however, be nullified by poor long-term glycemic control [19].

Therefore, if the therapy of neonatal diabetes is complex and at greater risk of severe hypoglycemia, on the other hand the risk of developing microvascular complications in the first 20 years of the disease remains limited and mainly associated with persistently high levels of glycated hemoglobin [17–19].

9.1.7 GLIS3

This syndrome is characterized by permanent neonatal diabetes and congenital hypothyroidism which can be mainly associated with intrauterine growth retardation, developmental delay, alterations in the renal, hepatic, and pancreatic exocrine parenchyma, glaucoma, facial dysmorphism, and abnormalities of the bone development.

In literature are reported 3 cases of deaths ranging in age from 6 months to 10 years, due to infectious complications (sepsis, pneumonia) in 3 out of 4 siblings belonging to the same family [20]. The same authors also identified two other families with a less severe phenotype.

In a larger case series, 12 cases with 2 deaths were reported. For the young age of the subjects described in the literature, there is insufficient information on the development of long-term complications [21].

However, based on the different phenotypic expressions in the known series, the possibility of developing: fibrosis and cirrhosis of the liver; bone malformations and fractures; intestinal malabsorption resulting from pancreatic insufficiency; difficulty in obtaining a good balance of thyroid hormone levels; various manifestations of poor glycemic control, such as extreme insulin sensitivity with recurrent hypoglycemia, significant glycemic variability, or insulin resistance.

9.1.8 NeuroG3

The mutation of this gene constitutes a rare finding (11 cases in the literature) described for the first time in 2006 [22] and is responsible for the failure to develop intestinal enteroendocrine cells with consequent congenital malabsorptive diarrhea; in a small number of cases, it is associated with permanent diabetes with neonatal onset or in more advanced pediatric age [23, 24].

The major complications are consequent to persistent diarrhea that occurs in the first week of life, which requires parenteral nutrition and can lead to growth retardation [25]; Two deaths were reported from complications following liver and bowel transplantation and from liver failure due to cholestasis secondary to parenteral nutrition.

9.1.9 NeuroD1

Heterozygous mutations in the NeuroD1 gene have previously been identified as the cause of a rare form of adult-onset monogenic diabetes (MODY 6). Recently *Rubio-Cabezas* et al. [26], presented two cases of permanent neonatal diabetes due to a homozygous mutation of the NeuroD1 gene. These patients were described with intrauterine growth retardation, learning difficulties, severe cerebellar hypoplasia, sensorineural deafness, and visual impairment due to severe myopia and retinal dystrophy.

A third case of neonatal diabetes induced by a different homozygous mutation of the same gene was identified by *Demirbilek H* et al. [27]. In this case, the patient presented poorly compensated diabetes, mental retardation, ataxic gait, inability to speak, clonic seizures, retinitis pigmentosa, sensorineural deafness, and cerebellar hypoplasia. The young age of the rare cases reported in the literature does not allow for information about the clinical evolution in adulthood. However, in the absence of good glycemic compensation, the development of micro and macrovascular complications for Type 1 diabetes is plausible.

9.1.10 PAX6

PAX6 is a transcription factor involved in eye and brain development and plays a role in pancreatic and pituitary development. In literature, a case of a patient with trisomy 21, microphthalmia, permanent neonatal diabetes, hypopituitarism, and a complex brain abnormality has been reported. It is described also that a brother, who died in infancy, had similar brain abnormalities, anophthalmia, and neonatal diabetes [28].

9.1.11 MNX1

MNX1 is known to be involved in caudal development and motor neuron differentiation and is the major susceptibility locus for dominant inherited sacral agenesis.

A homozygous mutation in the MNX1 gene was reported in 2013 by *Bonnefond A* et al. in a patient with diabetes onset at 17 days of life and a history of severe intrauterine developmental delay. The girl at 18 months still showed an insulin requirement of 0.8 U/kg/day [29].

In 2014 *Flanagan SE* et al. identified two other subjects where the MNX1 gene mutation was at the origin of neonatal diabetes and intrauterine growth retardation. In one of the two patients, there was also widespread extrapancreatic involvement with severe developmental delay, poor sucking and swallowing, neurogenic bladder, flexion deformity of the legs, short stature (lower third percentile), rocker feet, generalized reduction of cerebral myelin, renal hypoplasia, sacral agenesis, imperforate anus, and finally, hypoplastic carriers that led to death from respiratory failure at the age of 10 months [30].

9.1.12 STAT3

In 2014, *Flanagan SE* et al. published a short paper describing a novel monogenic cause of autoimmunity resulting from de novo germline activating STAT3 gene mutations in five individuals with a spectrum of early-onset autoimmune diseases [31]. These included 3 subjects with permanent neonatal diabetes associated with other autoimmune endocrinopathies and 1 subject with isolated permanent neonatal diabetes. In these patients, diabetes started in the first weeks of life (median 2.5 weeks, range 0–43 weeks) and had total endogenous insulin deficiency since diagnosis. Three of the four affected individuals had autoantibodies to pancreatic islets. The authors hypothesized that autoimmune beta-cell destruction began during fetal life, given the intrauterine growth retardation and early-onset of diabetes (≤3 weeks).

Additional associated autoimmune conditions included autoimmune enteropathy, autoimmune interstitial lung disease, juvenile arthritis, and primary hypothyroidism. Other common features were short stature and eczema.

9.1.13 NKX2-2

Recessive mutations in the NKX2-2 gene were reported in 2014 by *Flanagan SE* et al. as a new cause of neonatal diabetes in 3 subjects [30], that also had intrauterine growth retardation (IUGR), severe retardation of both motor and intellectual development, with hypotonia, cortical blindness, hearing and visual tracking impairment.

A further case was reported by *Auerbach A* et al. in a newborn with very low birth weight (VLBW) and neonatal diabetes (NDM), with severe obesity and developmental delay already at the age of 1 year [32]. Glycemic control was unexpectedly achieved with a regimen of 3 daily doses of slow insulin analogues, while severe obesity was associated with a paradoxical increase in postprandial ghrelin, as detected by an oral glucose tolerance test conducted at age of 3.5 years. For the rare causes of monogenic neonatal diabetes, the small number of cases in the literature is not sufficient to obtain precise information on the evolution of the clinical picture in later life. However, it is likely that the major complications are those deriving from the various and often severe diseases associated with neonatal diabetes, and that the latter, given the complete insulin dependence, may show a course comparable to that of Type 1 diabetes mellitus.

9.1.14 Wolfram Syndrome

Wolfram syndrome (WS) is a rare neurodegenerative disorder that is characterized by diabetes insipidus, diabetes mellitus, optic atrophy, and deafness [33]. WS is a progressive neurodegenerative disorder, which should always be suspected in patients with insulin-dependent diabetes and optic atrophy. Diabetic ketoacidosis is a rare complication, the insulin requirement is low with a clinical course not progressive and milder than Type 1 diabetes. Microvascular complications are uncommon, and they are likely related to residual insulin secretion. Unfortunately, hypoglycemia episodes may be frequent due to neurologic dysfunctions, which may lead to hypoglycemia unawareness [34].

Optic atrophy is characterized by a progressive decrease in visual acuity with a color vision defect, which leads to blindness. Less frequent findings may include cataract, nystagmus, and pigmentary retinopathy [34]. Moreover, other possible clinical findings that involve different organs may occur such as sensorineural hearing loss. The clinical spectrum may range from congenital deafness to mild impairment, which is sometimes progressive because of the central nervous system's degenerative process [35, 36]. Diabetes mellitus is not the only endocrine disease described in patients with WS. Diabetes insipidus is frequent too, and it occurs mostly in the second decade of life [37]. Furthermore, male patients may present hypogonadism more frequently than females, secondary to hypothalamus–pituitary axis impairment or gonadal failure. Hypothyroidism and growth retardation have also been reported [34]. Neurologic abnormalities are described and occur later in patients' life in about 60% of the patients. The neurologic abnormalities are progressive, leading to general brain atrophy, which is more prominent in the cerebellum, pons, and medulla, and there is brain stem and cranial nerve involvement [38–40].

References

1. Hattersley AT, Greeley SAW, Polak M, Rubio-Cabezas O, Njølstad PR, Mlynarski W, Castano L, Carlsson A, Raile K, Chi DV, Ellard S, Craig ME. ISPAD clinical practice consensus guidelines 2018: the diagnosis and management of monogenic diabetes in children and adolescents. Pediatr Diabetes. 2018 Oct;19(Suppl 27):47–63. https://doi.org/10.1111/pedi.12772.
2. Bacon S, Kyithar MP, Rizvi SR, Donnelly E, McCarthy A, Burke M, Colclough K, Ellard S, Byrne MM. Successful maintenance on sulphonylurea therapy and low diabetes complication rates in a HNF1A-MODY cohort. Diabet Med. 2016;33(7):976–84. https://doi.org/10.1111/dme.12992. Epub 2015 Nov 17

3. Delvecchio M, Pastore C, Giordano P. Treatment options for MODY patients: a systematic review of literature. Diabetes Ther. 2020;11(8):1667–85. https://doi.org/10.1007/s13300-020-00864-4. Epub 2020 Jun 24
4. Velho G, Blanché H, Vaxillaire M, Bellanné-Chantelot C, Pardini VC, Timsit J, Passa P, Deschamps I, Robert JJ, Weber IT, Marotta D, Pilkis SJ, Lipkind GM, Bell GI, Froguel P. Identification of 14 new glucokinase mutations and description of the clinical profile of 42 MODY-2 families. Diabetologia. 1997 Feb;40(2):217–24. https://doi.org/10.1007/s001250050666.
5. Steele AM, Shields BM, Wensley KJ, Colclough K, Ellard S, Hattersley AT. Prevalence of vascular complications among patients with glucokinase mutations and prolonged, mild hyperglycemia. JAMA. 2014 Jan 15;311(3):279–86. https://doi.org/10.1001/jama.2013.283980.
6. Murphy R, Ellard S, Hattersley AT. Clinical implications of a molecular genetic classification of monogenic beta-cell diabetes. Nat Clin Pract Endocrinol Metab. 2008;4(4):200–13. https://doi.org/10.1038/ncpendmet0778. Epub 2008 Feb 26
7. Isomaa B, Henricsson M, Lehto M, Forsblom C, Karanko S, Sarelin L, Häggblom M, Groop L. Chronic diabetic complications in patients with MODY3 diabetes. Diabetologia. 1998 Apr;41(4):467–73. https://doi.org/10.1007/s001250050931.
8. Ulinski T, Lescure S, Beaufils S, Guigonis V, Decramer S, Morin D, Clauin S, Deschênes G, Bouissou F, Bensman A, Bellanné-Chantelot C. Renal phenotypes related to hepatocyte nuclear factor-1beta (TCF2) mutations in a pediatric cohort. J Am Soc Nephrol. 2006;17(2):497–503. https://doi.org/10.1681/ASN.2005101040. Epub 2005 Dec 21
9. Bellanné-Chantelot C, Clauin S, Chauveau D, Collin P, Daumont M, Douillard C, Dubois-Laforgue D, Dusselier L, Gautier JF, Jadoul M, Laloi-Michelin M, Jacquesson L, Larger E, Louis J, Nicolino M, Subra JF, Wilhem JM, Young J, Velho G, Timsit J. Large genomic rearrangements in the hepatocyte nuclear factor-1beta (TCF2) gene are the most frequent cause of maturity-onset diabetes of the young type 5. Diabetes. 2005 Nov;54(11):3126–32. https://doi.org/10.2337/diabetes.54.11.3126.
10. Dubois-Laforgue D, Cornu E, Saint-Martin C, Coste J, Bellanné-Chantelot C, Timsit J. Monogenic diabetes study Group of the Société Francophone du Diabète. Diabetes, associated clinical Spectrum, long-term prognosis, and genotype/phenotype correlations in 201 adult patients with hepatocyte nuclear factor 1B (HNF1B) molecular defects. Diabetes Care. 2017;40(11):1436–43. https://doi.org/10.2337/dc16-2462. Epub 2017 Apr 18
11. Barbetti F, D'Annunzio G. Genetic causes and treatment of neonatal diabetes and early childhood diabetes. Best Pract Res Clin Endocrinol Metab. 2018;32(4):575–91. https://doi.org/10.1016/j.beem.2018.06.008. Epub 2018 Jun 25
12. Busiah K, Drunat S, Vaivre-Douret L, Bonnefond A, Simon A, Flechtner I, Gérard B, Pouvreau N, Elie C, Nimri R, De Vries L, Tubiana-Rufi N, Metz C, Bertrand AM, Nivot-Adamiak S, de Kerdanet M, Stuckens C, Jennane F, Souchon PF, Le Tallec C, Désirée C, Pereira S, Dechaume A, Robert JJ, Phillip M, Scharfmann R, Czernichow P, Froguel P, Vaxillaire M, Polak M, Cavé H, French NDM study group. Neuropsychological dysfunction and developmental defects associated with genetic changes in infants with neonatal diabetes mellitus: a prospective cohort study [corrected]. Lancet Diabetes Endocrinol. 2013;1(3):199–207. https://doi.org/10.1016/S2213-8587(13)70059-7. Epub 2013 Sep 6. Erratum in: Lancet Diabetes Endocrinol. 2013 Nov;1(3): e14
13. Beltrand J, Elie C, Busiah K, Fournier E, Boddaert N, Bahi-Buisson N, Vera M, Bui-Quoc E, Ingster-Moati I, Berdugo M, Simon A, Gozalo C, Djerada Z, Flechtner I, Treluyer JM, Scharfmann R, Cavé H, Vaivre-Douret L, Polak M, GlidKir Study Group. Sulfonylurea therapy benefits neurological and psychomotor functions in patients with neonatal diabetes owing to potassium channel mutations. Diabetes Care. 2015;38(11):2033–41. https://doi.org/10.2337/dc15-0837. Epub 2015 Oct 5. Erratum in: Diabetes Care. 2016 Jan;39(1):175
14. Bowman P, Sulen Å, Barbetti F, Beltrand J, Svalastoga P, Codner E, Tessmann EH, Juliusson PB, Skrivarhaug T, Pearson ER, Flanagan SE, Babiker T, Thomas NJ, Shepherd MH, Ellard S, Klimes I, Szopa M, Polak M, Iafusco D, Hattersley AT, Njølstad PR, Neonatal Diabetes

International Collaborative Group. Effectiveness and safety of long-term treatment with sulfonylureas in patients with neonatal diabetes due to KCNJ11 mutations: an international cohort study. Lancet Diabetes Endocrinol. 2018;6(8):637–46. https://doi.org/10.1016/S2213-8587(18)30106-2. Epub 2018 Jun 4. Erratum in: Lancet Diabetes Endocrinol 2018 Sep;6(9):e17

15. Bowman P, Broadbridge E, Knight BA, Pettit L, Flanagan SE, Reville M, Tonks J, Shepherd MH, Ford TJ, Hattersley AT. Psychiatric morbidity in children with KCNJ11 neonatal diabetes. Diabet Med. 2016;33(10):1387–91. https://doi.org/10.1111/dme.13135. Epub 2016 May 21
16. Svalastoga P, Sulen Å, Fehn JR, Aukland SM, Irgens H, Sirnes E, Fevang SKE, Valen E, Elgen IB, Njølstad PR. Intellectual disability in K_{ATP}Channel neonatal diabetes. Diabetes Care. 2020;43(3):526–33. https://doi.org/10.2337/dc19-1013. Epub 2020 Jan 13
17. Nordwall M, Fredriksson M, Ludvigsson J, Arnqvist HJ. Impact of age of onset, puberty, and glycemic control followed from diagnosis on incidence of retinopathy in type 1 diabetes: the VISS study. Diabetes Care. 2019;42(4):609–16. https://doi.org/10.2337/dc18-1950. Epub 2019 Jan 31
18. Hietala K, Harjutsalo V, Forsblom C, Summanen P, Groop PH, FinnDiane Study Group. Age at onset and the risk of proliferative retinopathy in type 1 diabetes. Diabetes Care. 2010;33(6):1315–9. https://doi.org/10.2337/dc09-2278. Epub 2010 Feb 25
19. Salardi S, Porta M, Maltoni G, Rubbi F, Rovere S, Cerutti F, Iafusco D, Tumini S, Cauvin V. Diabetes Study Group of the Italian Society of Paediatric Endocrinology and Diabetology. Infant and toddler type 1 diabetes: complications after 20 years' duration. Diabetes Care. 2012;35(4):829–33. https://doi.org/10.2337/dc11-1489. Epub 2012 Feb 8
20. Senée V, Chelala C, Duchatelet S, Feng D, Blanc H, Cossec JC, Charon C, Nicolino M, Boileau P, Cavener DR, Bougnères P, Taha D, Julier C. Mutations in GLIS3 are responsible for a rare syndrome with neonatal diabetes mellitus and congenital hypothyroidism. Nat Genet. 2006;38(6):682–7. https://doi.org/10.1038/ng1802. Epub 2006 May 21
21. Dimitri P, Habeb AM, Gurbuz F, Millward A, Wallis S, Moussa K, Akcay T, Taha D, Hogue J, Slavotinek A, Wales JK, Shetty A, Hawkes D, Hattersley AT, Ellard S, De Franco E. Expanding the Clinical Spectrum Associated With GLIS3 Mutations. J Clin Endocrinol Metab. 2015;100(10):E1362–9. https://doi.org/10.1210/jc.2015-1827. Epub 2015 Aug 10. Erratum in: J Clin Endocrinol Metab. 2015 Dec;100(12):4685. Garbuz, F [corrected to Gurbuz, F]
22. Wang J, Cortina G, Wu SV, Tran R, Cho JH, Tsai MJ, Bailey TJ, Jamrich M, Ament ME, Treem WR, Hill ID, Vargas JH, Gershman G, Farmer DG, Reyen L, Martín MG. Mutant neurogenin-3 in congenital malabsorptive diarrhea. N Engl J Med. 2006;355(3):270–80. https://doi.org/10.1056/NEJMoa054288.
23. Germán-Díaz M, Rodriguez-Gil Y, Cruz-Rojo J, Charbit-Henrion F, Cerf-Bensussan N, Manzanares-López Manzanares J, Moreno-Villares JM. A new case of congenital Malabsorptive diarrhea and diabetes secondary to mutant Neurogenin-3. Pediatrics. 2017;140(2):e20162210. https://doi.org/10.1542/peds.2016-2210.
24. Solorzano-Vargas RS, Bjerknes M, Wang J, Wu SV, Garcia-Careaga MG, Pitukcheewanont P, Cheng H, German MS, Georgia S, Martín MG. Null mutations of NEUROG3 are associated with delayed-onset diabetes mellitus. JCI Insight. 2020;5(1):e127657. https://doi.org/10.1172/jci.insight.127657.
25. Pinney SE, Oliver-Krasinski J, Ernst L, Hughes N, Patel P, Stoffers DA, Russo P, De León DD. Neonatal diabetes and congenital malabsorptive diarrhea attributable to a novel mutation in the human neurogenin-3 gene coding sequence. J Clin Endocrinol Metab. 2011;96(7):1960–5. https://doi.org/10.1210/jc.2011-0029. Epub 2011 Apr 13
26. Rubio-Cabezas O, Minton JA, Kantor I, Williams D, Ellard S, Hattersley AT. Homozygous mutations in NEUROD1 are responsible for a novel syndrome of permanent neonatal diabetes and neurological abnormalities. Diabetes. 2010;59(9):2326–31. https://doi.org/10.2337/db10-0011. Epub 2010 Jun 23
27. Demirbilek H, Hatipoglu N, Gul U, Tatli ZU, Ellard S, Flanagan SE, De Franco E, Kurtoglu S. Permanent neonatal diabetes mellitus and neurological abnormalities due to a novel

homozygous missense mutation in NEUROD1. Pediatr Diabetes. 2018;19(5):898–904. https://doi.org/10.1111/pedi.12669. Epub 2018 Mar 27
28. Solomon BD, Pineda-Alvarez DE, Balog JZ, Hadley D, Gropman AL, Nandagopal R, Han JC, Hahn JS, Blain D, Brooks B, Muenke M. Compound heterozygosity for mutations in PAX6 in a patient with complex brain anomaly, neonatal diabetes mellitus, and microophthalmia. Am J Med Genet A. 2009;149A(11):2543–6. https://doi.org/10.1002/ajmg.a.33081.
29. Bonnefond A, Vaillant E, Philippe J, Skrobek B, Lobbens S, Yengo L, Huyvaert M, Cavé H, Busiah K, Scharfmann R, Polak M, Abdul-Rasoul M, Froguel P, Vaxillaire M. Transcription factor gene MNX1 is a novel cause of permanent neonatal diabetes in a consanguineous family. Diabetes Metab. 2013;39(3):276–80. https://doi.org/10.1016/j.diabet.2013.02.007. Epub 2013 Apr 4
30. Flanagan SE, De Franco E, Lango Allen H, Zerah M, Abdul-Rasoul MM, Edge JA, Stewart H, Alamiri E, Hussain K, Wallis S, de Vries L, Rubio-Cabezas O, Houghton JA, Edghill EL, Patch AM, Ellard S, Hattersley AT. Analysis of transcription factors key for mouse pancreatic development establishes NKX2-2 and MNX1 mutations as causes of neonatal diabetes in man. Cell Metab. 2014;19(1):146–54. https://doi.org/10.1016/j.cmet.2013.11.021.
31. Flanagan SE, Haapaniemi E, Russell MA, Caswell R, Allen HL, De Franco E, McDonald TJ, Rajala H, Ramelius A, Barton J, Heiskanen K, Heiskanen-Kosma T, Kajosaari M, Murphy NP, Milenkovic T, Seppänen M, Lernmark Å, Mustjoki S, Otonkoski T, Kere J, Morgan NG, Ellard S, Hattersley AT. Activating germline mutations in STAT3 cause early-onset multi-organ autoimmune disease. Nat Genet. 2014;46(8):812–4. https://doi.org/10.1038/ng.3040. Epub 2014 Jul 20
32. Auerbach A, Cohen A, Ofek Shlomai N, Weinberg-Shukron A, Gulsuner S, King MC, Hemi R, Levy-Lahad E, Abulibdeh A, Zangen D. NKX2-2 mutation causes congenital diabetes and infantile obesity with paradoxical glucose-induced ghrelin secretion. J Clin Endocrinol Metab. 2020;105(11):dgaa563. https://doi.org/10.1210/clinem/dgaa563.
33. Wolfram DJ, Wagener HP. Diabetes mellitus and simple optic atrophy among siblings: report of four cases. Mayo ClinProc. 1938;13:715–8.
34. Delvecchio M, Iacoviello M, Pantaleo A, Resta N. Clinical Spectrum associated with Wolfram syndrome type 1 and type 2: a review on genotype-phenotype correlations. Int J Environ Res Public Health. 2021;18(9):4796. https://doi.org/10.3390/ijerph18094796.
35. Pennings RJ, Huygen PL, van den Ouweland JM, Cryns K, Dikkeschei LD, Van Camp G, Cremers CW. Sex-related hearing impairment in Wolfram syndrome patients identified by inactivating WFS1 mutations. Audiol Neurootol. 2004;9(1):51–62. https://doi.org/10.1159/000074187.
36. Karzon R, Narayanan A, Chen L, Lieu JEC, Hershey T. Longitudinal hearing loss in Wolfram syndrome. Orphanet J Rare Dis. 2018 Jun 27;13(1):102. https://doi.org/10.1186/s13023-018-0852-0.
37. Fonseca SG, Ishigaki S, Oslowski CM, Lu S, Lipson KL, Ghosh R, Hayashi E, Ishihara H, Oka Y, Permutt MA, Urano F. Wolfram syndrome 1 gene negatively regulates ER stress signaling in rodent and human cells. J Clin Invest. 2010;120(3):744–55. https://doi.org/10.1172/JCI39678. Epub 2010 Feb 15
38. Barrett TG, Bundey SE, Macleod AF. Neurodegeneration and diabetes: UK nationwide study of Wolfram (DIDMOAD) syndrome. Lancet. 1995 Dec 2;346(8988):1458–63. https://doi.org/10.1016/s0140-6736(95)92473-6.
39. Pakdemirli E, Karabulut N, Bir LS, Sermez Y. Cranial magnetic resonance imaging of Wolfram (DIDMOAD) syndrome. Australas Radiol. 2005 Apr;49(2):189–91. https://doi.org/10.1111/j.1440-1673.2005.01420.x.
40. Domenech E, Gomez-Zaera M, Nunes V. Wolfram/DIDMOAD syndrome, a heterogenic and molecularly complex neurodegenerative disease. Pediatr Endocrinol Rev. 2006 Mar;3(3):249–57.

GPSR Compliance

The European Union's (EU) General Product Safety Regulation (GPSR) is a set of rules that requires consumer products to be safe and our obligations to ensure this.

If you have any concerns about our products, you can contact us on ProductSafety@springernature.com

In case Publisher is established outside the EU, the EU authorized representative is:

Springer Nature Customer Service Center GmbH
Europaplatz 3
69115 Heidelberg, Germany

Batch number: 10370712

Printed by Printforce, the Netherlands